Cancer Update:
Current topics in research

Cancer Update:
Current topics in research

Based on an international educational seminar held in
Tokyo on July 15–16, 1989

Editors: **Tetsuo Taguchi**
Emil Frei III

 1990

Excerpta Medica, Amsterdam–Princeton–Hong Kong–Tokyo–Sydney

Current Clinical Practice Series No. 58
ISBN 90 219 1790 4

This publication has been made possible through a grant from Taiho Pharmaceutical Co., Ltd., Tokyo, Japan.

Publisher: Excerpta Medica

Offices: P.O. Box 1126   15-23, Nishi-Azabu 4-chome
               1000 BC Amsterdam   Minato-ku, Tokyo

               P.O. Box 3085   M.L.C. Centre, Level 49
               Princeton, N.J. 08540   Martin Place, Sydney 2000

               67 Wyndham Street
               Hong Kong

Printed in Japan

Organizing Committee

Advisors: Tamaki Kajitani
Japanese Foundation for Cancer Research

Kiyoji Kimura
National Nagoya Hospital and Nagoya Memorial Hospital

Organizers: Tetsuo Taguchi
Research Institute for Microbial Diseases, Osaka University

Setsuo Fujii
The Osaka Foundation for Promotion of Fundamental Medical Research

Program Committee Members:

Kazuo Ota
Nagoya Memorial Hospital

Hisashi Furue
Teikyo University

Hisanobu Niitani
Nippon Medical School

Shigeru Tsukagoshi
Cancer Chemotherapy Center, Japanese Foundation for Cancer Research

Hisashi Majima
Ichijokai Hospital

Contents

Preface

With changes in society, culture, and lifestyle, diseases are becoming more and more complicated and diverse. Cancer is no exception. We have to study not only the disease itself, but also increasingly wider fields including the effects of surgery, radiotherapy, and chemotherapy, as well as the quality of life.

It was an honor and a pleasure to have been able to hold such a symposium as "Cancer Update," with eminent physicians in the field of cancer therapy from the USA reviewing the most up-to-date knowledge and achievements.

I have always been interested in and had great respect for the planning and programs of the Educational Symposia of the American Society of Clinical Oncology (ASCO). The programs are more thorough each year and I am always impressed by their timeliness. I had been thinking that it would be useful if more physicians from Japan could attend such seminars. That was why I suggested a seminar like the ASCO Educational Symposia when Taiho Pharmaceutical Co., Ltd., was considering what type of event to hold in commemoration of the 5th anniversary of the launch of tegafur. They agreed with my idea and asked me to organize the symposium.

Dr Setsuo Fujii, who developed tegafur, joined me as co-organizer of the meeting. We also asked Drs Tamaki Kajitani and Kiyoji Kimura to act as advisors and Drs Kazuo Ota, Hisashi Furue, Hisanobu Niitani, Shigeru Tsukagoshi, and Hisashi Majima to become program committee members. Although ASCO's seminars are excellent, we could not directly reproduce them in Japan and we had many discussions before we eventually completed the final program. Looking back, I am quite satisfied that the meeting sustained the spirit of ASCO's Educational Symposia. I am also very pleased that, in addition to the seminar, we also had a panel discussion with all the presenting physicians as panelists and Drs Tsukagoshi and Majima as chairpersons.

The seminar, held on July 15–16, 1989, was a great success, with 600 delegates attending, thanks to the 8 physicians from the USA and all those who contributed to its organization. I would like to express my sincere thanks to all those concerned and also to Mr Kobayashi, President of Taiho Pharmaceutical Co., Ltd.

Lastly, I would also like to express my deepest regret at the loss of Dr Setsuo Fujii, who died on August 4, 1989. We will cherish his memory always.

Tetsuo Taguchi, M.D.
Professor and Chairman
Department of Oncologic Surgery
Research Institute for Microbial Diseases
Osaka University
Osaka, Japan

Preface

Surgery and radiotherapy will cure 30–40% of patients who develop cancer. Most of the rest die because of systemic tumor, ie, metastases. The successful treatment of micro- or macrometastatic disease must be systemic.

In 1947, Farber introduced the first successful treatment of leukemia and Rhodes introduced the nitrogen mustards in 1945 and 1946. These early temporary successes prompted a major investment in cancer chemotherapy. New agents were discovered and by the mid- and late 1960s, the principles of therapeutic research in cancer were established. This included such clinical variables as dose, schedule, and combination and sequential therapy. The proper application of these principles led to the curative treatment first of acute lymphocytic leukemia, then of Hodgkin disease and non-Hodgkin lymphoma, for testis cancer, and for some of the childhood solid tumors.

In 1970 the curative intent focus shifted to adjuvant chemotherapy. This occurred primarily because of the recognition that microscopic tumor deposits are much more readily eradicated by chemotherapy than macroscopic disease. Initially in breast cancer and osteogenic sarcoma, it was demonstrated that adjuvant chemotherapy was substantially effective, decreasing mortality by 25% in premenopausal patients with breast cancer and some 60–70% in patients with osteogenic sarcoma. More recently, the use of adjuvant chemotherapy in the form of fluorouracil plus levamisole has decreased mortality in patients with the appropriate stage of colorectal cancer.

Finally, neoadjuvant chemotherapy was developed in an effort to reduce and render more operable selected solid tumors. In addition, neoadjuvant chemotherapy provided systemic treatment up front, which is ideal, based on our knowledge of clonal evolution to drug resistance. Neoadjuvant chemotherapy has proven effective in head and neck cancer, stage III breast cancer, invasive bladder cancer, and other selected diseases. While tumor regression has been achieved in a major way in these programs, survival improvement has not yet been demonstrated.

Perhaps the most compelling reality of modern cancer therapeutic research is related to the impact of the rapid advances in molecular biology and immunology. Increasingly, such findings are being applied to clinical material. Oncogenes and oncogene products, such as growth factors, can be secreted by tumor cells, often interacting with adjacent normal cells to maintain the malignant phenotype. Indeed, there are circumstances where a tumor cell produces a growth factor and also a surface receptor for the growth factor, allowing for autocrine maintenance of the neoplastic state. Molecular biological products such as tumor necrosis factor, the interferons, and hematopoietins will have a significant effect on therapy today and increasingly in the immediate future. The control of transcription, such as with antisense compounds, may also control the neoplastic phenotype. The ability to identify such an oncogene product that, for example, has enzymatic activity, allows for the application of crystallography, X ray diffraction, and computer graphing of the 3-dimensional enzyme, followed by selected site synthesis of analogues.

It has been estimated that information and concepts relating to basic tumor biology are doubling every 7 years. Such advances cannot help but have a profound positive impact in the clinic in the immediate and long-range future. This cancer update thus serves the very important role of bringing to the physicians the expanding and changing body of knowledge that is cancer.

Emil Frei III, M.D.
Director and Physician-in-Chief
Dana-Farber Cancer Institute
Boston, Massachusetts, USA

Special lecture I

Biochemical strategy of cancer cells and enzyme-pattern-targeted chemotherapy

George Weber

Laboratory for Experimental Oncology and Walther Oncology Center, Indiana University School of Medicine, Indianapolis, Indiana

Introduction

Cancer is the second most common cause of death in the USA and it is a major clinical and biological problem. An understanding of the biochemical differences between normal and cancer cells should provide paradigms for problem solving in cancer research and yield approaches in the rational design of chemotherapy. Studies carried out in my laboratory with guidance of the molecular correlation concept identified important aspects of the biochemical strategy of cancer cells [1,2]. The approach adopted by our laboratory is indicated in Table 1.

Table 1 Biochemical basis of cancer chemotherapy.

1) Transformation	Commitment to continued replication
	Biochemical program of quantitative imbalance
2) Progression	Escalation in expression of neoplasia; growth and spread
	Amplification of quantitative and qualitative biochemical imbalance
3) Drug treatment	Should interfere with the biochemical program of the commitment to replication and cause selective cell death

Biochemical basis of cancer chemotherapy

In the biochemistry of cancer cells there are transformation- and progression-linked alterations. In the progression of the cancer cells there is an escalation in the expression of neoplastic properties and, correspondingly, an amplification of the quantitative and qualitative biochemical differences which distinguish cancer cells from normal ones [2]. Drug treatment should interfere only with the biochemical program of the commitment to replication and it should cause selective

3

death of the cancer cells. The host cells should adapt and recover from toxicity. The biochemical studies have revealed operation of gene logic in cancer cells. The following will illuminate the operation of gene logic in pyrimidine and purine metabolism in cancer cells which forms the basis for antimetabolite chemotherapy. It will also underline the international nature of cancer research carried out in my laboratory.

Pyrimidine metabolic imbalance in cancer cells

An outstanding aspect of gene logic is the reciprocal regulation of the activities of key enzymes and metabolic pathways [1,2]. The operation of reciprocal regu-

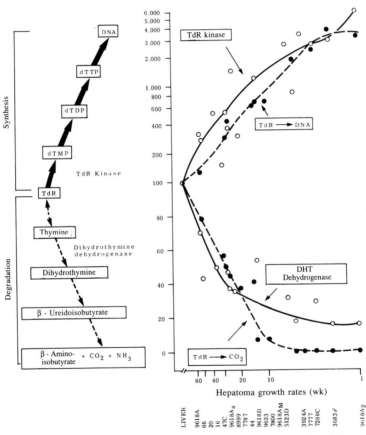

Fig 1 Reciprocal behavior of activities of opposing key enzymes, thymidine (TdR) kinase and dihydrothymine (DHT) dehydrogenase (assayed in cytoplasmic extracts), and of synthetic and catabolic pathways of thymidine (measured in tissue slices by the incorporation of thymidine into DNA and by the degradation of thymidine to CO$_2$). Activities were expressed as percentages of values of liver of control normal rats. Heavy lines indicate the enzymic activities that were increased and broken lines the activities that were decreased.

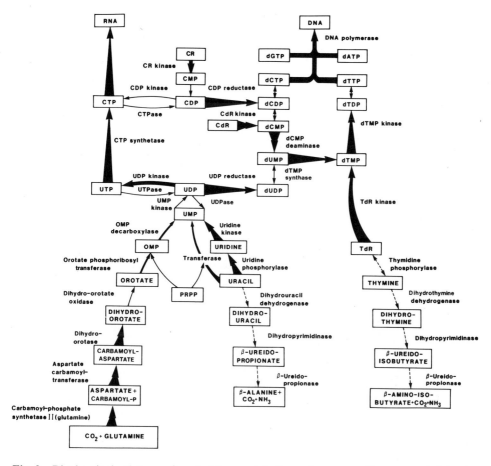

Fig 2 Biochemical strategy of pyrimidine metabolism of cancer cells as revealed in the integrated reprogramming of gene expression manifested in the imbalance of activities of key enzymes of de novo and salvage biosynthetic and degradative pathways. Tapered, thick arrows, enzymic activities that are increased with tumor proliferative rate (progression-linked alterations); broken arrows, enzymic activities that are decreased; straight thick arrows (eg, UDP kinase, orotidine-5'-monophosphate decarboxylase), enzymic activities that are increased in all the tumors (transformation-linked); dotted straight arrows, (eg, thymidine phosphorylase), enzymic activities that are decreased in all the neoplasms. Arrows with normal thinness, no relation found with transformation and progression (eg, dihydroorotate oxidase) or the behavior has not yet been determined (eg, CDP kinase). Heavy lines indicate the enzymic activities that were increased and broken lines the activities that were decreased.

lation was first shown in carbohydrate metabolism in our laboratory in 1968 [3]. Reciprocal regulation in thymidine metabolism was demonstrated by Japanese and American colleagues (Figs 1 and 2) [1,2,4,5]. As shown in Fig 1, thymidine metabolism involves its utilization to DNA and its degradation to CO_2. Thymidine kinase channels thymidine to DNA biosynthesis and its action is opposed by the rate-limiting enzyme of degradation, dihydrothymine dehydrogenase. Dr Taiichi Shiotani, then working in my laboratory, now at Kagawa University, showed that thymidine kinase activity was elevated in all examined rat hepatomas and it progressively increased in slow, intermediate, and rapidly growing hepatomas [4]. Concurrently, as shown by Dr Sherry Queener, dihydrothymine dehydrogenase activity decreased in these tumors [6]. The first isolation of dihydrothymine dehydrogenase was also accomplished by Shiotani [7]. Dr John Ferdinandus showed that not only was the enzymic equilibrium altered in these hepatomas but, as measured in tissue slices, thymidine incorporation to DNA increased; by contrast, thymidine degradation, as indicated by the release of CO_2, declined [8]. This is an example of reciprocal regulation of the activities of antagonistic pathways of synthesis and degradation in cancer cells. There is strong parallelism between the behavior of the activities of the key enzymes and those of the overall pathways.

The overall de novo biosynthesis of DNA progresses through the increased activities of key enzymes into dUMP and then to DNA. In the cancer cells in the overall pyrimidine metabolic imbalance, the synthetic enzyme activities were elevated, whereas those of degradation were decreased. In the de novo UMP biosynthesis, the activities of the key enzymes increased; concurrently, the enzymes of uridine degradation decreased [2].

Selective advantages and chemotherapeutic targeting

This altered enzymic balance amplifies the biochemical alterations and confers selective advantages to cancer cells. In identifying these selective advantages we can pinpoint the enzymes against which chemotherapy should be directed. Therefore, it is an important matter to identify such potential target enzymes [2].

The first and rate-limiting enzyme of UMP biosynthesis is carbamoyl phosphate synthase II. Dr Takashi Aoki of Juntendo University, working in my laboratory, showed that synthase II activity increased in all tumors (transformation-linked) and gradually increased in the intermediate and rapidly growing hepatomas (progression-linked alteration) (Fig 3) [9]. There are a number of such transformation- and progression-linked increased enzymic activities in de novo DNA biosynthesis and they have been used as clinical targets of cancer drug treatment.

Relationship of de novo and salvage activities: clinical implications

The specific activities of the key enzymes of de novo pyrimidine biosynthesis are low, whereas those of the salvage enzymes are high (Fig 4) [2]. This relationship of de novo and salvage activities has an important implication for clinical chemotherapy. The following example should illuminate the significance of these relationships (Figs 4 and 5).

In dTMP biosynthesis the rate-limiting enzyme is ribonucleotide reductase.

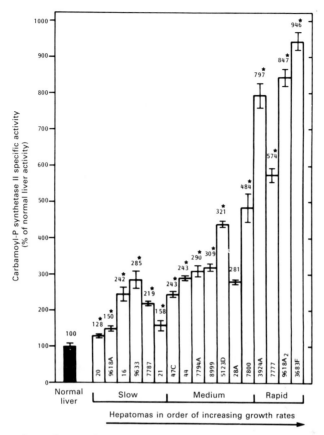

Fig 3 The transformation- and progression-linked behavior of the activity of carbamoyl-phosphate synthase II in hepatomas of different growth rates. Mean specific activities (± SE) are plotted as percentages of normal liver value. Asterisks indicate values significantly different from that of the normal liver (p<0.05).

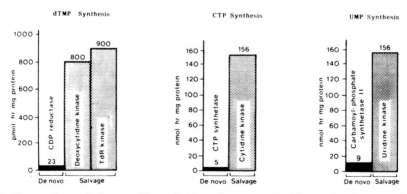

Fig 4 Comparison of the specific activities of the rate-limiting and salvage pyrimidine enzymes involved in the synthesis of dTMP (left), CTP (middle), and UMP (right) in normal rat liver. TdR, thymidine.

When, in clinical treatment, this enzyme is inhibited by hydroxyurea, the block of DNA biosynthesis may not be complete because the activity of the salvage enzyme, deoxycytidine kinase, is much higher and it may circumvent the block. Furthermore, thymidine kinase activity is also higher than that of the reductase and this salvage enzymic activity also may circumvent the inhibition of the reductase activity. When 5-fluorouracil (5FU) or methotrexate is administered in the clinic to inhibit the activity of dTMP synthase, thymidine kinase salvage activity can circumvent this block. This biochemical relationship is significant in clinical treatment as it explains, in part at least, the weak and undependable action of 5FU in carcinoma of the colon where it causes temporary remissions in 20% of cases. In spite of these remissions, the end result is usually the same whether or not 5FU is used. The reason for this chemotherapeutic failure is the overlooking of the presence of high salvage thymidine kinase activity in human colon tumors [10,11]. For better chemotherapeutic success, inhibitors of thymidine uptake, eg, dipyridamole, or inhibitors of thymidine kinase should be used in combination chemotherapy (Fig 5) [2]. The same situation applies to CTP biosynthesis. When the rate-limiting enzyme CTP synthase is inhibited in the tumor cells by an antiglutamine agent, eg, acivicin, the activity of cytidine kinase can circumvent the block of CTP biosynthesis (Fig 5) [2]. The same argument applies to blockers of key enzymes of de novo UMP biosynthesis. If synthase II activity is inhibited by an antiglutamine agent, uridine kinase can circumvent the block. If N-phosphonoacetyl-L-aspartate (PALA) is used, uridine kinase and/or uracil phosphoribosyltransferase activity can overcome the inhibition of UMP biosynthesis (Fig 5). It is therefore essential to combine inhibitors of enzymes of de novo pathway with blockers of the salvage pathways [2].

Purine metabolic imbalance in cancer cells

The enzymic imbalance in purine metabolism of cancer cells is shown in Fig 6. Dr Nobuhiko Katunuma, a visiting professor in my department, first showed that the activity of amidophosphoribosyltransferase, the first and rate-limiting enzyme of de novo purine biosynthesis, increased in rat hepatomas [12]. Continuing this work, Dr Noemi Prajda, from Hungary, demonstrated that this enzymic activity was elevated 2- to 3-fold in all hepatomas, whether they were of slow, intermediate, or rapid growth rates, and was transformation-linked [13]. Katunuma, with Dr Michio Tsuda, now at Tokai University, isolated the enzyme from a rapidly growing rat hepatoma [14]. Subsequently, Prajda determined that the rate-limiting enzyme of the degradation of IMP, xanthine oxidase, was markedly decreased in all hepatomas in a transformation-linked fashion [15]. In consequence, there is an increased capacity in these tumors to synthesize IMP and a marked decline in the capacity to degrade it. This is the operation of reciprocal regulation in purine metabolism. In consequence, there is an overwhelming capacity in cancer cells to make IMP that can be channeled to the

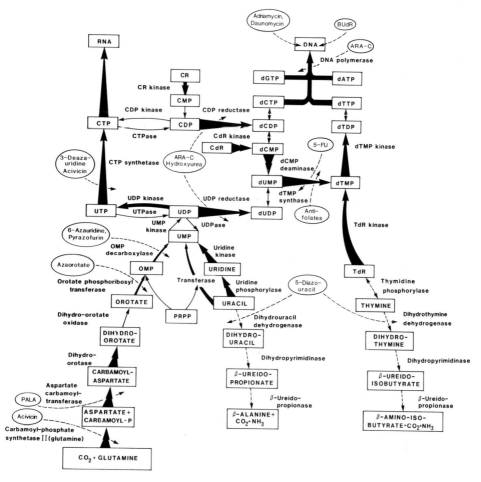

Fig 5 Pyrimidine metabolic imbalance in cancer cells and key enzymes as targets of anti-cancer clinical and experimental drugs. It is clear that enzymes of de novo pathways are targets and the activities of the salvage enzymes can circumvent the blocks as indicated. BUdR, bromodeoxyuridine; ARA-C, 1-ß-D-arabino-furanosylcytosine; CR, cytidine; CdR, deoxycytidine; OMP, orotidine 5'-monophosphate.

biosynthesis of adenylates or guanylates.

The interconversion of purines and the enzymic utilization of IMP were examined in my laboratory in detail by Dr Robert C. Jackson, from the UK, and Theodore Boritzki. Our earliest investigations carried out in this area showed that the activity of IMP dehydrogenase (IMP DH), the rate-limiting enzyme of GTP biosynthesis, increased in all the hepatomas in parallel with the growth rate [16]. Thus, IMP DH is a transformation- and progression-linked enzyme (Fig 7). We also reported that GMP synthase activity was elevated [17] and that there was an increase in the concentration of GMP and dGTP in hepatomas [18]. Therefore,

9

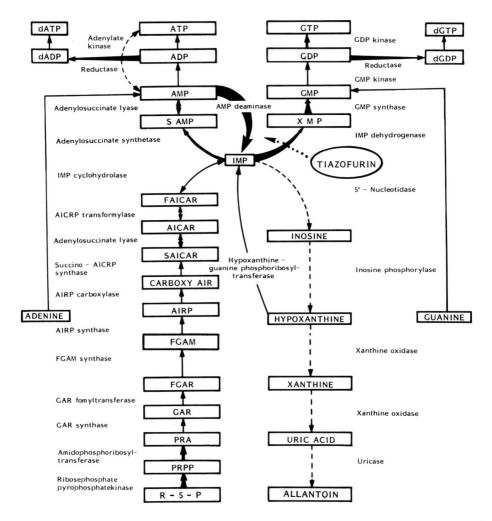

Fig 6 Biochemical strategy for purine metabolism of cancer cells as revealed in the integrated reprogramming of gene expression manifested in the imbalance of the activities of key enzymes of de novo and salvage biosynthesis and of the degradative pathway.

it appeared that the overall capacity for GTP biosynthesis is up-regulated in cancer cells. Similar increased enzymic activities of the guanylate biosynthetic enzymes were observed for other types of solid tumors in animals and humans and also in human leukemia.

Selective advantages and targeting of antipurine chemotherapy

An increased guanylate biosynthetic capacity should confer selective advantages to cancer cells and therefore this pathway should be a sensitive target to chemo-

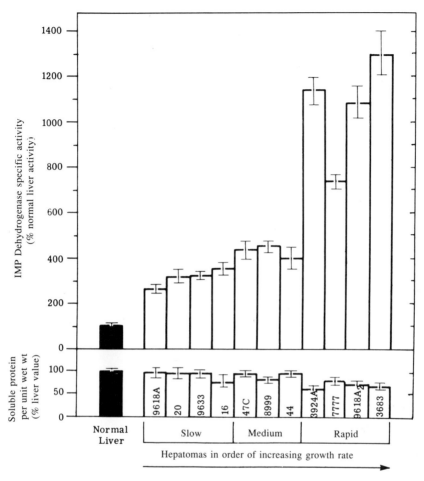

Fig 7 Transformation- and progression-linked increase in the behavior of the activity of IMP DH in hepatomas of different growth rates. Mean specific activities (± SE) are plotted as percentages of the normal liver values. All hepatoma activities were significantly higher than those of the normal liver (p<0.05).

therapy. We singled out the increased activity of IMP DH as a potentially sensitive target because this enzyme has the lowest activity among all the enzymes of purine metabolism [19].

Relations between purine de novo and salvage pathways

In recent years Dr Yutaka Natsumeda of Yokohama University, working in my laboratory, made new observations indicating that the activities of the purine salvage enzymes, adenine phosphoribosyltransferase and hypoxanthine-guanine phosphoribosyltransferase, were markedly higher than those of the key enzymes of the biosynthesis of AMP, IMP, or GMP (Fig 8) [20]. We also observed that the affinity of the salvage enzymes to PRPP was much better than that of amidophosphoribosyltransferase, the rate-limiting purine biosynthetic enzyme [2,20]. The clinical relevance of this is that in cancer chemotherapy, inhibition of key enzymes of purine de novo biosynthesis is not an adequate treatment measure, because the high activities of the salvage enzymes of cancer cells can circumvent the block of purine biosynthesis [2]. However, there are no good inhibitors of the purine salvage enzymes. We provided evidence that dipyridamole, an inhibitor of the transport of salvage precursors, provides synergism with blockers of enzymes of de novo purine biosynthesis [2].

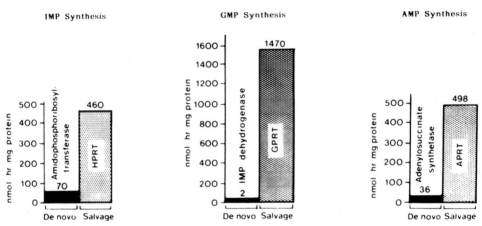

Fig 8 Comparison of the specific activities of the rate-limiting and salvage purine enzymes involved in the synthesis of IMP (left), GMP (middle), and AMP (right) in normal liver.

Tiazofurin, an inhibitor of IMP DH

We had previously emphasized that the elevated activity of IMP DH, the rate-limiting enzyme of de novo GTP biosynthesis, should be a sensitive target in the design of anticancer chemotherapy [2,19,21,22]. Dr Roland K. Robins, one of the foremost synthetic chemists in the USA, at that time at the University of Utah, took up our suggestion [23] and produced a number of compounds for inhibition of IMP DH, including ribavirin, an antiviral drug, and tiazofurin (2-ß-D-ribofuranosylthiazole-4-carboxamide, NSC 286193) [23], a C-nucleoside, which proved to be of interest in this action against neoplastic cells, including murine tumors [24–27]. Investigations revealed that tiazofurin is a prodrug that must be converted into thiazole-4-carboxamide adenine dinucleotide (TAD) to yield a powerful inhibition of IMP DH activity at concentrations of 10^{-7} M [24–27]. As shown in Fig 9, in sensitive cells tiazofurin is converted, through the action of 2 enzymes, to TAD, an analog of NAD; TAD can be broken down by a phosphodiesterase to inactive compounds. It was shown that murine tumors that

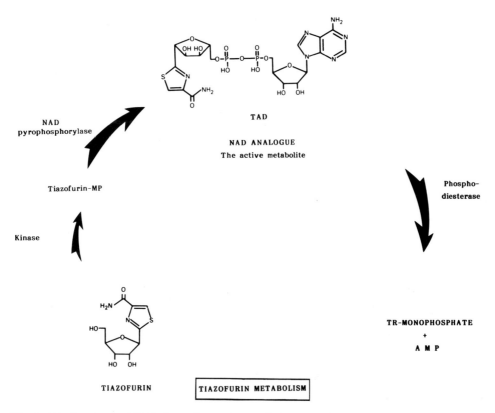

Fig 9   Biochemistry of TAD formation and degradation.

produced high concentrations of TAD were sensitive to the antitumor action of tiazofurin, whereas if they did not, the tumors proved to be resistant to this drug. However, in phase I/II clinical trials in patients with solid tumors, at the US National Cancer Institute (NCI) and 10 other centers, reports of side effects, chiefly neurotoxicity [28], have restricted the progress of studies of this drug in humans.

Our new approach: use of tiazofurin in clinical treatment of leukemia

Our studies in hepatoma-bearing rats showed that a single ip injection of tiazofurin rapidly lowered IMP DH activity and, subsequently, the concentrations of guanylates. These parameters returned to preinjection levels within 24–36 h [29]. The growth of the subcutaneously implanted hepatomas was inhibited by tiazofurin treatment. This new evidence brought a reexamination of the clinical results. I concluded that the clinical trials could be greatly improved and the biochemical impact of tiazofurin could be monitored in leukemic patients where serial sampling of the neoplastic cells would be feasible.

13

Evidence that tiazofurin should be effective in leukemia

Earlier murine studies indicated the effectiveness of tiazofurin in P388 and L1210 leukemias. However, the clinical studies were carried out in patients with solid tumors because progress seemed to be needed most in those neoplastic diseases [28] and tiazofurin was not tested in leukemics. In collaboration with my clinical colleagues at Indiana University in Indianapolis, we tested samples and found evidence that IMP DH activity in human leukemic cells was 20- to 40-fold higher than in normal leukocytes [30]. It was a matter of concern, however, that the activity of the guanylate salvage enzyme, guanine phosphoribosyltrans-ferase (GPRT), in normal leukocytes was 100-fold higher than that of IMP DH and the GPRT activity was increased further (2- to 6-fold) in the leukemic leukocytes (Table 2) [30]. Additional investigations revealed that when labeled tiazofurin was incubated with normal or leukemic leukocytes, the leukemic leukocytes produced 20- to 30-fold more TAD than the normal ones (Table 3)

Table 2 Purine enzymic program in normal and leukemic leukocytes.

	De novo: IMP DH nmol/h/mg protein	%	Salvage: GPRT nmol/h/mg protein	%
Normal	31.5 ± 0.5	100	389 ± 27	100
Leukemic patients				
1[*]	47.7 ± 0.4	1539[†]	1101 ± 12	283[†]
2[††]	80.8 ± 0.8	2606[†]	1766 ± 21	454[†]
3[§]	129.0 ± 5.4	4161[†]	2653 ± 12	682[†]

(Mean $\pm$ SE of 3 to 9 assays).
[*]Acute megakaryoblastic leukemia; [†]significantly higher than normal leukocytes (p<0.05); [††]blast crisis of CML; [§]acute mixed myeloid-lymphoid leukemia.

Table 3 Production of TAD from tiazofurin in leukocytes from healthy volunteers and leukemic patients. Reprinted, with permission, from Jayaram HN et al [31].

	No. of patients	TAD pmol/10^9 cells/h	% Normal
Normal	5	27 ± 8	100
Acute nonlymphocytic leukemia	9	551 ± 71	2040
Acute lymphoblastic leukemia	3	756 ± 94	2800

Bone marrow cells were 90–99% blasts and were obtained from patients 3–14 months after last treatment.

[31]. On the basis of this and other evidence (Table 4), we obtained approval for a phase I/II trial in which we proposed to decrease tiazofurin toxicity by infusing the drug daily for a 1-h period, using a pump to achieve an even flow and repeatability. This method replaced the one used earlier by the NCI and other centers, which involved a 10-min bolus or continuous infusion [32]. Our protocol specified end-stage leukemic patients, with emphasis on chronic myelogenous leukemia in blast crisis. Our treatment schedule is outlined in Table 5.

Table 4 Evidence that human myelocytic leukemia should be a sensitive target for treatment with tiazofurin.

1) IMP DH activity in myelocytic leukemia cells was markedly elevated above that of normal leukocytes
2) On incubation with tiazofurin TAD accumulated in leukemic leukocytes above that observed in normal bone marrow cells
3) On incubation with tiazofurin in leukemic cells from bone marrow or peripheral blood the GTP concentration decreased; there was no change in normal granulocytes
4) In previous phase I studies with solid tumors, mild myelosuppression was observed
5) In kinetic studies the IMP DH activity was strongly inhibited by TAD in concentrations that proved to be available in the blast cells of patients

Table 5 Treatment schedule with tiazofurin.

1) Tiazofurin was started at 2200 mg/m^2
2) IMP DH activity and GTP concentrations were measured 3 × per day
3) All patients received allopurinol to decrease uric acid production
4) Adequate biochemical response:
   a. 80% decline in GTP pools;
   b. 90% decrease in IMP DH activity
5) Tiazofurin was escalated with 1100 mg/m^2 in case of inadequate biochemical response after 2–5 days of treatment
6) Adequate dose of tiazofurin was given for 5–15 days based on biochemical and hematologic response

Our clinical results in sensitive leukemic patients indicated that tiazofurin infusion was successful in rapidly lowering IMP DH activity in mononuclear cells ($t_{\frac{1}{2}} = 30$ min) and subsequently the GTP concentration declined ($t_{\frac{1}{2}} = 2$–3 days). These biochemical events were followed by the decline and clearing of blast cells from the circulation. In contrast, the granulocyte counts were maintained and not depleted and neutropenia did not occur when the patients were treated with daily infusions for 15 days or less (Fig 10) [22,30,33,34].

15

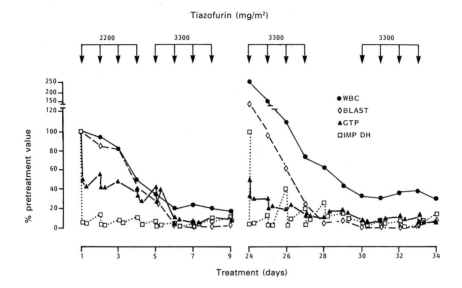

Fig 10 Changes in hematological and biochemical parameters during 2 consecutive courses of tiazofurin treatment in patient no. 4. The values of WBC, blast cells, GTP pools, and IMP DH activity are expressed as a percentage of pretreatment values. The pretreatment value of WBC was 6.6×10^9/L; blast cells, 4.0×10^9/L; GTP pools, 344.3 nmol/10^9 leukemic cells; and IMP DH activity, 12.2 nmol/h/mg protein.

Inhibition of salvage guanylate synthesis by hypoxanthine

Our protocol specified allopurinol treatment (300 mg/day) to decrease uric acid production. This dose was successful in curtailing plasma uric acid level; however there was a steady see-sawing of the serum hypoxanthine concentration. After the patient received the allopurinol pill in the morning, hypoxanthine concentration increased, but within a few hours it declined [34,35]. We carried out studies on the effect of hypoxanthine and observed that it competitively inhibited GPRT activity. Then we established that it was necessary to increase the serum hypoxanthine concentration to at least 60 μM in order to decrease the salvage activity to less than 10%. The behavior of plasma tiazofurin levels and hypoxanthine concentrations, as well as the biochemical response to tiazofurin, are shown in Fig 11.

Our objective was to produce a high concentration of plasma hypoxanthine and achieve a plateau around 40–60 μM. Figure 12 shows that we achieved this in a 22-year-old leukemic patient and subsequently in other cases.

16

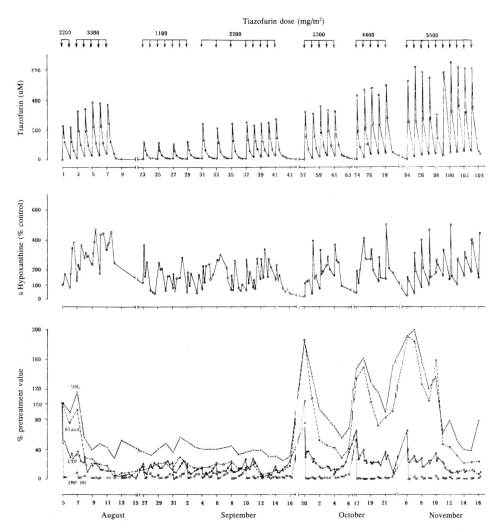

Fig 11 Treatment of a patient showing plasma tiazofurin and hypoxanthine concentrations and the biochemical and clinical impact of the drugs. In this early treatment protocol, 1 pill of 300 mg allopurinol was given in the mornings.

Clinical summary of response by July 1989

A survey of the first 16 cases indicated that tiazofurin achieved a 50% response rate in these patients and nearly all chronic granulocytic leukemia (CGL) patients in blast crisis responded well. The duration of response was from 1 to 10 months and survival was 1–16 months (Table 6) [34]. Current studies, on the first 24 patients, confirmed these observations [35].

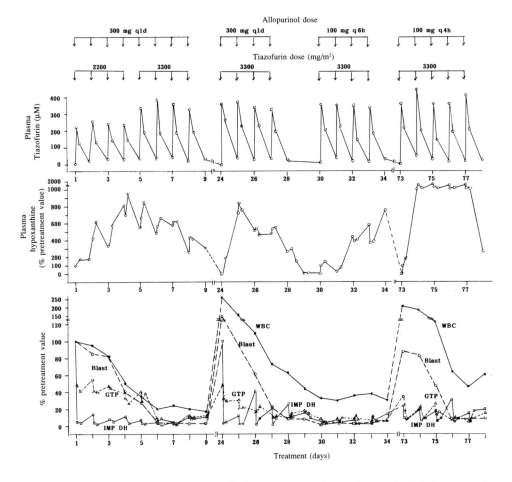

Fig 12 Treatment of a patient with tiazofurin and changes in the dose and administration of allopurinol. Behavior of plasma tiazofurin and hypoxanthine concentrations is shown with the biochemical and hematological impact of the drugs.

Evidence for tiazofurin-induced in vivo differentiation

Examination of differential bone marrow smears before and after tiazofurin treatment indicated that cellularity was maintained, the blast cells decreased, and the mature forms of mononuclear cells increased (Table 7) [33,34]. Previous in vitro studies found that addition of tiazofurin resulted in a decrease in GTP concentration and in induced differentiation in HL-60 cells in tissue culture [37,38]. However there was no evidence that these events were reproduced in vivo in animals or humans. Our results, therefore, appear to be the first to show in vivo differentiation in patients produced by tiazofurin [33,34]. We attribute the main-

Table 6 Patient characteristics, total dose, and number of days of intial tiazofurin treatment, outcome, and duration of response.

Patient	Sex/Age (y)	Disease	Status	Total dose of tiazofurin (mg/m²)	No. of days	Outcome	Response duration (mo)	Total survival (mo)
Responders								
1	F/53	ANLL	First relapse	19 000	7	Complete remission	10	15
2	M/27	CGL	Myeloid blast crisis	41 800	11	Complete remission	3	4
3	F/20	CGL	Myeloid blast crisis	22 000	8	Complete response	6	6*
4	M/44	CGL	Myeloid blast crisis	24 200	11	Complete response	7	13
5	M/56	CGL	Myeloid blast crisis	46 200	6	Complete response	6	13
6	F/58	CGL	Myeloid blast crisis	20 900	7	Hematologic improvement	10	16
7	M/70	ANLL	Secondary leukemia	33 000	9	Antileukemic effect	<1	<1
8	M/55	ANLL	First relapse	89 100	26	Antileukemic effect	<1	<1
Nonresponders								
9	M/48	ANLL	Second relapse	23 650	11	No response		4
10	F/21	ANLL	Second relapse	49 500	18	No response		2
11	F/37	ANLL	Refractory	52 500	20	No response		<1
12	M/24	ANLL	First relapse	27 500	10	No response		2
13	M/41	ANLL	First relapse	20 900	10	No response		6
Unevaluable for hematological effect								
14	M/83	ANLL	Post MDS	14 300	5	Unevaluable		<1
15	F/50	ANLL	Post MDS	5 500	3	Unevaluable		8
16	M/27	CGL	Myeloid blast crisis	2 200	1	Unevaluable		<1

ANLL, acute nonlymphocytic leukemia; CGL, chronic granulocytic leukemia.
*Patient returned to primary physician in California, who treated her with mitoxanthrone to prepare her for bone transplantation, but the patient died during mitoxanthrone chemotherapy.

Table 7 Differential of bone marrows before and after tiazofurin treatment in patients with good response.

No.	Cellularity*		Blasts		Pro + Myelo		MM + Gran	
	Before	After	Before	After	Before	After	Before	After
1	Hypo	Normal	36	0	0	15	22	78
2	Hyper	Hyper	25	5	14	0	45	74
3	Hyper	Hyper	NE[†]	NE				
4	Hyper	Hyper	55	10	29	47	0	40
5	Hyper	Hypo	33	2	28	20	38	54
6	Hyper	Normal	48	2	8	14	41	72
7	Hyper	Hyper	74	17	6	36	17	37
8	Hyper	Hyper	60	1	12	6	5	93
9	Normal	Hypo	82	0	1	0	10	0

Pro, promyelocytes; Myelo, myelocytes; MM, metamyelocytes; Gran, granulocytes.
*Cellularity estimated in bone marrow biopsies or aspirates.
[†]Not evaluable due to dry tap.

tenance of bone marrow cellularity to the fact that normal mononuclear cells produced only low concentrations of TAD from tiazofurin [31].

Tiazofurin down-regulates oncogenes in K562 cells and in hepatoma 3924A cells in culture

New light was thrown on the possible mechanisms of induced differentiation at the molecular level in our studies in K562 human erythroleukemic cells. When K562 cells were cultured in the presence of tiazofurin (10 μM), the IMP DH activity and GTP concentration decreased, followed by a down-regulation of the c-Ki-*ras* oncogene and a subsequent emergence of induced differentiation [39]. Evidence was found that the c-*myc* oncogene was also down-regulated [39]. If the cascade is the same or similar in leukemic cells during tiazofurin treatment, then this may well be the first instance of cancer chemotherapeutic action of a drug due to down-regulation of an oncogene in patients. That this down-regulation of oncogenes by tiazofurin is not restricted to leukemic cells was shown in our recent studies where the c-*myc* and the c-Ha-*ras* gene expression was down-regulated by tiazofurin in rat hepatoma 3924A cells [40]. Therefore, since tiazofurin in vitro and in leukemic patients caused induced differentiation of leukemic cells, the impact of the drug in hepatoma cells and in leukemic patients might be exerted, in part at least, through a down-regulation of the *myc* and *ras* oncogenes. Thus, the action of tiazofurin might have a cascade of triple impact: 1) chemotherapy; 2) down-regulation of oncogenes; and 3) induced differentiation (Fig 13).

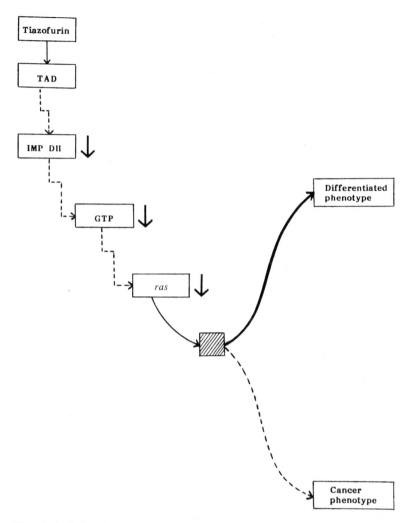

Fig 13 Tiazofurin-induced cascade in sensitive cells. Tiazofurin is converted into TAD which inhibits IMP DH activity, leading to the decrease of GTP concentration. The low GTP concentration limits the expression of the *ras* oncogene which suppresses the expression of the cancer phenotype and allows the emergence of a differentiated phenotype.

Biochemically targeted and monitored chemotherapy trial

On the basis of the principles discussed above, enzyme-pattern-targeted chemo-therapy of leukemia was designed. Tiazofurin was targeted against the increased IMP DH activity to control de novo biosynthesis in leukemic cells. Allopurinol, originally included in the protocol to decrease serum uric acid concentration, was now also utilized to raise plasma hypoxanthine concentration to inhibit GPRT

21

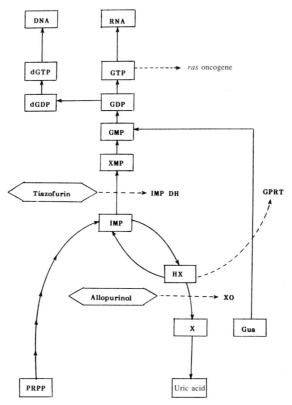

Fig 14 Impact of tiazofurin on primary (IMP DH), secondary (GTP), and tertiary (*ras* oncogene) targets. Allopurinol treatment inhibits liver xanthine oxidase activity and increases plasma hypoxanthine level which should inhibit the activity of the salvage enzyme GPRT.

activity and to inhibit the guanine salvage (Fig 14). Our approach, devised with collaborators Drs Guido J. Tricot and Ronald Hoffman of the Division of Hematology/Oncology in the Department of Medicine and Drs H.N. Jayaram and Y. Natsumeda in the Laboratory for Experimental Oncology, provides a number of advantages over the conventional chemotherapy of end-stage leukemia.

Conventional antileukemic treatment has several drawbacks.

1) Current treatment of leukemia is nonselective and profoundly affects normal hematopoietic and other rapidly dividing cells.

2) No rapid and convenient predictive in vitro tests are available to assess sensitivity to the drugs to be used.

3) No techniques are available to monitor chemotherapeutic action during treatment.

4) In relapsed patients, the effect of antileukemic drugs decreases markedly, but toxicity remains the same.

5) There is a 15–25% mortality due to treatment in newly diagnosed patients; the mortality is higher in refractory ones.

The following biochemical and clinical rationales support the testing of tiazofurin treatment of human leukemia, as also based on our observations made in the phase I/II trials at this university [33–35].

1) There is enzymic evidence for the up-regulation of the capacity for GTP production in human myelocytic leukemic cells as evidenced by increased activities of IMP DH and GMP synthase over the activities observed in normal leukocytes.

2) An in vitro predictive test is available to determine the sensitivity to tiazofurin of leukemic cells. Leukemic cells produce 20-fold higher concentrations of TAD from tiazofurin than normal leukocytes; as a result the GTP pool decreases in the leukemic leukocytes, whereas there is little change in the normal ones.

3) The high activity of the salvage enzyme GPRT in the leukemic cells is apparently curtailed by the low concentrations of guanine in the blood.

4) Allopurinol administration increases plasma hypoxanthine concentration, which competitively inhibits GPRT activity and thus decreases guanine salvage.

5) Samples of the leukemic and normal leukocyte population are readily available from peripheral blood and in most cases from the bone marrow in sufficient quantity to carry out the biochemical assays.

6) Measurement of the impact of tiazofurin on the targets, IMP DH activity and GTP concentration in the blast cells, makes it possible to measure the extent and duration of the drug action and to monitor the hematologic response.

7) Our schedule of administering tiazofurin in a 60-min infusion, using a pump to achieve uniform delivery, has markedly decreased toxicity, particularly neurotoxicity, that occurred in the earlier regimens of other investigators who used bolus injection of 10 min × 5 or continuous infusion for 5 days.

8) With resources to measure IMP DH activity, GTP and TAD concentration in the mononuclear cells, and tiazofurin and hypoxanthine levels in the plasma, it has been possible to achieve effective treatment in over 50% of cases, with low toxicity and good quality of life. A number of the clinical and biochemical aspects of this protocol and the prevention and treatment of side effects require further careful investigation.

Novel aspects of the tiazofurin treatment program for leukemia are summarized in Table 8.

Table 8   Novel aspects of tiazofurin treatment of refractory leukemia.

1) Rational targeting: IMP DH, GTP
2) Biochemistry provides monitoring during therapy
3) Selective to leukemic cells
4) Predictive test available
5) Induces differentiation
6) Does not produce neutropenia
7) Lowers toxicity
8) Avoids morbidity and mortality of conventional chemotherapy

The current treatment protocol uses 2200–4400 mg/m^2 tiazofurin over a period of 15 days or less. After 3 weeks the treatment can be repeated. An important feature of this trial is that once the dose is adjusted it is not necessary to escalate in the subsequent relapses and the patient can be kept at the same tiazofurin level for many cycles. This insight for obviation of the need to escalate at each relapse was achieved by measuring the response to tiazofurin of the targets, IMP DH activity and GTP concentration. This enzyme-pattern-targeted chemotherapy may therefore serve as a paradigm for other cancer drug treatment schedules where measurement of the biochemical targets of the drugs may well eliminate the need for escalation of drug treatment at each relapse.

A further advantage of our treatment relates to our observation that the resistance to tiazofurin frequently develops only after many months of drug administration. In some of these patients who had been completely resistant to hydroxyurea and 6-thioguanine, it became feasible after our tiazofurin treatment to reintroduce these drugs, when the patients were found to be highly sensitive to them. Whether we are dealing here with a reversal of multidrug resistance or with a new clone that has never been exposed to hydroxyurea or 6-thioguanine is under investigation.

The studies presented indicate the usefulness of the understanding of the biochemical differences between normal and cancer cells in the design and monitoring of enzyme-pattern-targeted chemotherapy of cancer.

Acknowledgments

These studies were supported by an Outstanding Investigator Grant CA-42510 from the National Cancer Institute, NIH, USPH.

References

1. Weber G. Enzymology of cancer cells. New Engl J Med 1987;296:486–93 & 541–51.
2. Weber G. Biochemical strategy of cancer cells and the design of chemotherapy: G.H.A. Clowes Memorial Lecture. Cancer Res 1983;43:3466–92.
3. Weber G. Carbohydrate metabolism in cancer cells and the molecular correlation concept. Naturwissenschaften 1968;55:418–29.
4. Weber G, Kizaki H, Shiotani T, et al. Biochemical strategy of hepatomas. J Toxicol Environ Hlth 1979;5:371–86.
5. Weber G, Queener SF, Ferdinandus JA. Control of gene expression in carbohydrate, pyrimidine and DNA metabolism. Adv Enzyme Regul 1971;9:63–95.
6. Queener SF, Morris HP, Weber G. Dihydrouracil dehydrogenase activity in normal, differentiating and regenerating liver and in hepatomas. Cancer Res 1971;31:1004–9.
7. Shiotani H, Weber G. Purification and properties of dihydrothymine dehydrogenase from rat liver. J Biol Chem 1981;256:219–24.
8. Ferdinandus JA, Morris HP, Weber G. Behavior of opposing pathways of thymidine

utilization in differentiating, regenerating and neoplastic liver. Cancer Res 1971;31: 550–6.

9. Aoki T, Morris HP, Weber G. Regulatory properties and behavior of activity of carbamoyl-phosphate synthetase II (glutamine-hydrolyzing) in normal and proliferating tissues. J Biol Chem 1982;257:432–8.

10. Denton J, Lui MS, Aoki T, et al. Enzymology of pyrimidine and carbohydrate metabolism in human colon carcinomas. Cancer Res 1982;42:1176–83.

11. Weber G, Ichikawa S, Nagai M, Natsumeda Y. Azidothymidine inhibition of thymidine kinase and synergistic cytotoxicity with methotrexate and 5-fluorouracil in rat hepatoma and human colon cancer cells. Cancer Commun 1990;2:129–33.

12. Katunuma N, Weber G. Glutamine phosphoribosylpyrophosphate amidotransferase: Increased activity in hepatomas. FEBS Lett 1974;49:53–6.

13. Prajda N, Katunuma N, Morris HP, Weber G. Imbalance of purine metabolism in hepatomas of different growth rates as expressed in behavior of glutamine PRPP amidotransferase (amidophosphoribosyltransferase, EC 2.4.2.14). Cancer Res 1975;35:3061–8.

14. Tsuda M, Katunuma N, Morris HP, Weber G. Purification, properties and immunotitration of hepatoma glutamine phosphoribosylpyrophosphate amidotransferase (amidophosphoribosyltransferase, EC 2.4.2.14). Cancer Res 1979;39:305–11.

15. Prajda N, Morris HP, Weber G. Imbalance of purine metabolism in hepatomas of different growth rates as expressed in behavior of xanthine oxidase (EC 1.2.3.2). Cancer Res 1976;36:4639–46.

16. Jackson RC, Weber G, Morris HP. IMP dehydrogenase, an enzyme linked with proliferation and malignancy. Nature 1975;256:331–3.

17. Boritzki TJ, Jackson RC, Morris HP, Weber G. Guanosine 5'-phosphate synthetase and guanosine 5'-phosphate kinase in rat hepatomas and kidney tumors. Biochim Biophys Acta 1981;658:102–10.

18. Jackson RC, Lui MS, Boritzki TJ, et al. Purine and pyrimidine nucleotide patterns of normal, differentiating and regenerating liver and of hepatomas in rats. Cancer Res 1980;40:1286–91.

19. Weber G, Prajda N, Jackson RC. Key enzymes of IMP metabolism: Transformation- and proliferation-linked alterations in gene expression. Adv Enzyme Regul 1976;14:3–24.

20. Natsumeda Y, Prajda N, Donohue JP, et al. Enzymic capacities of purine de novo and salvage pathways for nucleotide synthesis in normal and neoplastic tissues. Cancer Res 1984;44:2475–9.

21. Weber G, Natsumeda Y, Pillwein K. Targets and markers of selective action of tiazofurin. Adv Enzyme Regul 1985;24:45–65.

22. Weber G. Critical issues in chemotherapy with tiazofurin. Adv Enzyme Regul 1989;29: 75–95.

23. Robins RK. Nucleoside and nucleotide inhibitors of inosine monophosphate (IMP) dehydrogenase as potential antitumor inhibitors. Nucleosides Nucleotides 1982;1:35–44.

24. Cooney DA, Jayaram HN, Glazer RI, et al. Studies on the mechanism of action of tiazofurin metabolism to an analog of NAD with potent IMP dehydrogenase-inhibitory activity. Adv Enzyme Regul 1983;21:271–303.

25. Earle MF, Glazer RI. Activity and metabolism of 2-ß-D-ribofuranosylthiazole-4-carboxamide in human lymphoid tumor cells in culture. Cancer Res 1983;43:133–7.

26. Jayaram HN, Dion RL, Glazer RI, et al. Initial studies on the mechanism of action of a new oncolytic thiazole nucleoside, 2-ß-D-ribofuranosylthiazole-4-carboxamide (NSC-286193). Biochem Pharmacol 1982;31:2371–80.

27. Robins RK, Srivastava PC, Narayanan VL, et al. 2-ß-D-Ribofuranosylthiazole-4-car-

boxamide, a novel potential antitumor agent for lung tumors and metastases. J Med Chem 1982;25:107–8.

28. O'Dwyer PJ, Shoemacher DD, Jayaram HN, et al. Tiazofurin, a new antitumor agent. Invest New Drugs 1984;2:79–84.

29. Lui MS, Faderan MA, Liepnieks JJ, et al. Modulation of IMP dehydrogenase activity and guanylate metabolism by tiazofurin (2-ß-D-ribofuranosylthiazole-4-carboxamide). J Biol Chem 1984;259:5078–82.

30. Weber G, Jayaram HN, Lapis E, et al. Enzyme-pattern-targeted chemotherapy with tiazofurin and allopurinol in human leukemia. Adv Enzyme Regul 1988;27:405–33.

31. Jayaram HN, Pillwein K, Nichols CR, et al. Selective sensitivity to tiazofurin of human leukemic cells. Biochem Pharmacol 1986;35:2029–32.

32. O'Dwyer PJ, King SA, Hoth DF, Leyland-Jones B. Tiazofurin, a review of the clinical and biochemical effects of an inosine monophosphate dehydrogenase inhibitor. In press

33. Tricot GJ, Jayaram HN, Nichols CR, et al. Hematological and biochemical action of tiazofurin in a case of refractory acute myeloid leukemia. Cancer Res 1987;47:4988–91.

34. Tricot GJ, Jayaram HN, Nichols CR, et al. Biochemically directed therapy of leukemia with tiazofurin, a selective blocker of inosine 5'-phosphate dehydrogenase activity. Cancer Res 1989;49:3696–701.

35. Tricot G, Jayaram HN, Weber G, Hoffman R. Tiazofurin: biological effects and clinical uses. Int J Cell Cloning 1990;8:161–70.

36. Weber G, Yamaji Y, Olah E, et al. Clinical and molecular impact of inhibition of IMP dehydrogenase activity by tiazofurin. Adv Enzyme Regul 1989;28:335–56.

37. Lucas DL, Webster HK, Wright DG. Purine metabolism in myeloid precursor cells during maturation. J Clin Invest 1983;72:1889–990.

38. Sokoloski JA, Blair OC, Sartorelli AC. Alterations in glycoprotein synthesis and guanosine triphosphate levels associated with the differentiation of HL-60 leukemia cells produced by inhibitors of inosine 5'-phosphate dehydrogenase. Cancer Res 1986;46:2314–9.

39. Olah E, Natsumeda Y, Ikegami T, et al. Induction of erythroid differentiation and modulation of gene expression by tiazofurin in K-562 leukemia cells. Proc Natl Acad Sci USA 1988;85:6533–7.

40. Olah E, Kote Z, Natsumeda Y, et al. Down-regulation of c-*myc* and c-Ha-*ras* gene expression by tiazofurin in rat hepatoma cells. Cancer Biochem Biophys 1990;11:107–17.

Discussion

Chairperson: **Yoshio Sakurai**

Dr Shigeru Tsukagoshi (Cancer Chemotherapy Center, Japanese Foundation for Cancer Research, Tokyo): You mentioned that there were some responders and nonresponders in the clinical trials with tiazofurin and you stressed the importance of inhibition of IMP dehydrogenase. Is it possible that, in the respondents, the effect can be attributed to inhibition of IMP dehydrogenase or are the pharmacokinetics more important? Could we possibly predict clinical responses from IMP dehydrogenase in tumors?

Dr Weber: It seems that the most predictive so far, with limited experience, is whether or not the patient's leukemic cells from the bone marrow or periphery produce large amounts of TAD. The sensitive ones produce a lot of TAD. In each relapse if the cells retain the capacity to convert tiazofurin to TAD, IMP dehydrogenase is decreased and the patient responds and goes into remission. Those who produced little TAD, and we have taken every consecutive patient without selection, were still treated, but there was poor response. So apparently the predictive test is useful and those patients who do not produce sufficient TAD do not respond. This is the basis for the nonresponders at present (Tricot G et al. Cancer Res 1989;49:3693–3701; Weber G. Adv Enzyme Regul 1989;29:75–95).

Dr Yoshio Sakurai (Kyoritsu College of Pharmacy, Tokyo): Is it a general phenomenon that malignant cells have high nucleoside salvage?

Dr Weber: Yes, all tumor cells we looked at had stepped-up salvage activity (Weber G. Cancer Res 1983;43:3466–92). There is particularly high salvage activity in colorectal cancer, which explains, in part, the difficulties in treating until we have good inhibitors of the salvage enzymes. It is a challenge for the synthetic chemist to provide selective inhibitors for thymidine kinase, uridine-cytidine kinase, deoxycytidine kinase, adenine phosphoribosyltransferase, and guanine-hypoxanthine phosphoribosyltransferase, because these 5 salvage enzymes would have to be inhibited. There are clinical studies ongoing with inhibitors of de novo pathways and dipyridamole. Dipyridamole blocks the transport into cells of the salvage precursors and in vitro it has been effective in providing synergism with blockers of the de novo synthetic pathways. In all human tumors we have looked at, salvage plays an important role (Weber G. Cancer Res 1983;43:3466–92; Weber G et al. Cancer Commun 1990;2:129–33.).

Dr Sakurai: Do you have any typical tumor models, for instance, a rodent tumor, the growth of which is retarded markedly only by blocking the salvage route?

Dr Weber: One model that we have been using is the Morris hepatoma series and hepatoma 3924A, which also is available in tissue culture. This tumor can be inhibited and in tissue culture the cells can be killed by combinations of an antiglutamine agent and dipyridamole (Zhen Y-S et al. Cancer Res 1983;43:1616–9), by methotrexate and dipyridamole, and by a number of inhibitors of de novo pathways and dipyridamole. If we had specific inhibitors for the salvage enzymes, we would have a more rational and effective chemotherapy.

Dr Masaichi Yamamura (Tokai University School of Medicine, Isehara): Supposing we could predict that a patient was not going to respond, would you treat this patient?

Dr Weber: Our idea with the predictive test is that eventually we can identify the patients who would not benefit from the therapy and those whom we would not recommend for treatment. Now we are testing the predictive test itself, whether it is dependable enough. At the moment the method we use is 85% predictive, so that it requires more experience before it could definitely predict that this patient should benefit and the other would not. At the moment, under the protocol, we have to test everybody and take every consecutive step, regardless of the result of the predictive test.

Dr Yamamura: Did you find any patients who did respond when the test predicted that they should not?

Dr Weber: Yes, we had 1 or 2 false positives and 1 or 2 false negatives, so we cannot say yet that this test is perfect in any way. We are testing the test itself, but it may be that we can use it to separate the population of patients who cannot respond from those who should respond. So far, in 85% of cases we obtained the clinical response that we predicted.

Special lecture II

Dose—A critical factor in cancer chemotherapy

Emil Frei III, Karen H. Antman, John Clark

Dana-Farber Cancer Institute, Boston, Massachusetts

Introduction

Dose is an important integral part of the strategy for cancer treatment. A steep dose-response curve with respect to both host and tumor in essentially all experimental, in vivo, and in vitro systems has been demonstrated. A major problem with those experimental systems was the high proliferative thrust. At a clinical level major progress in acute lymphocytic leukemia was made over a period of 10 years. That progress depended upon numerous innovations involving experimental design and the development of supportive care [1,2]. The first issue that had to be addressed, in terms of chemotherapy, was the production of complete remission. At that time (1955–65), we had single agents, including 2 antimetabolites, vincristine and prednisone, all of which were capable of producing complete remission in a few patients. With combinations of 2 agents, such as methotrexate and 6-mercaptopurine, a disappointingly low complete response rate of 45% was achieved. However, when we used agents with differing dose-limiting toxicity such as vincristine and prednisone in such a way that they could be combined at full dose, complete remission rates of 90% were achieved. This was the first clinical evidence that dose was important. Unfortunately, all of the patients who entered complete remission relapsed and we therefore needed to direct our investigations toward the question of treatment during complete remission. Patients were randomly allocated to full-dose or half-dose therapies, and treatment was maintained during remission. In this circumstance, ie, against minimal disease, there was a highly significant difference in terms of duration of remission in favor of the high dose [3]. Thus, not only for remission induction against overt disease, but also against microscopic disease, dose was a major determinant of response. When this had been accomplished and with treatment of the pharmacologic sanctuary, ie, the central nervous system, acute lymphocytic leukemia was converted from an incurable disease to a disease that was curable in about 50% of patients. This was shown in studies started in the late 1960s and early 1970s (Fig 1) [1].

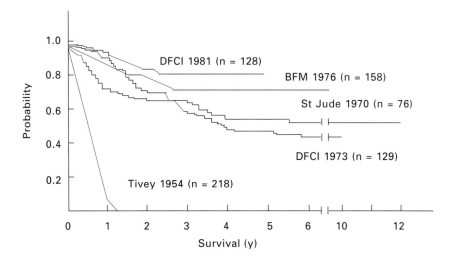

Fig 1   Survival of schoolchildren with acute lymphocytic leukemia.

With the realization that chemotherapy was more than palliative, at least for acute leukemia, we began to appreciate certain basic tenets that were important in the construction of clinical trials. A neoplastic event affects one normal cell in the body. That cell is rendered neoplastic and undergoes proliferative (clonal) expansion. If all of the cancer cells were derived from a single normal cell, one would expect cancers to be highly homogeneous. We know from almost every science (immunology, chemotherapy, and cytogenetics) that cancers, particularly in the advanced form, are highly heterogeneous. With time, with mitotic history, aneuploidy occurs, increasing cell death, drug resistance, and decreasing growth fraction, all of which are adverse with respect to the implications of systemic treatment: chemotherapy, immunotherapy, or hormonal treatment [4].

The following illustrates 1 example of heterogeneity with respect to chemotherapy. Four cell lines were established from a human metastatic melanoma. Two of the cell lines were highly sensitive to the agent carmustine (BCNU) and 2 were highly resistant to the same agent. Such heterogeneity indicates multiple targets and the need for multiple-targeted therapy, ie, therapy that involves combinations of agents. With that realization, and particularly with the experience in acute lymphocytic leukemia, the next disease we challenged was Hodgkin's disease.

By 1963 we had 4 agents for Hodgkin's disease (Table 1). All 4 had the major limitation of producing complete remission in only a few patients. However, when they were put together in the well-known MOPP (mechlorethamine, vincristine sulfate, procarbazine, and prednisone) program, it was possible to use full doses of 2 of the agents and 60% full doses of 2 of the remaining agents.

Table 1 Hodgkin's disease: MOPP.

Drug(s)	Dose-limiting toxicity	% Full dose	Response (%)	
			PR & CR	CR
HN$_2$	Marrow	100	55	10
Vincristine	Neuropathy	100	60	5
Prednisolone	Steroid	100	35	5
Procarbazine	Marrow	100	60	15
MOPP	—	60–100–100–60		70
				(50% cure)

Dose was then maintained. With this combination the complete response rate was now 70% and the cure rate 50% [5,6]. Figure 2 represents an NCI update of the MOPP program. The disease-free survival plateau is now at 50–60% and extends over more than 20 years. As with acute lymphocytic leukemia, there has been a marked and continuing reduction in mortality from Hodgkin's disease in the USA.

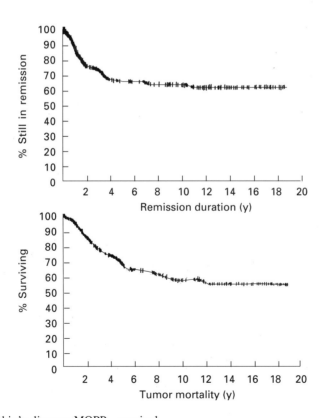

Fig 2 Hodgkin's disease: MOPP—survival.

33

The cure of cancer by chemotherapy requires that you have 3 or more active agents (Table 2). The following formula provides a good generalization in preparing a curative chemotherapy strategy. If you use these agents in combination and use them in circumstances where there is minimal compromise in dose, cure may occur. Tumor burden is inversely related to curability. This is clearly true for the diseases discussed above, but these are the rapidly moving diseases. What about the much more common, slower-moving tumors such as breast, lung, and colon cancers? This brings us to the role of adjuvant chemotherapy.

Table 2 Curative chemotherapy strategy.

$$\text{Cure} \propto \frac{\text{Active agents } (3+)^{(a)} \times \text{combinations}^{(a)} \times \text{dose}^{(b)}}{\text{Tumor burden}^{(c)} \times \text{prior therapy}^{(d)}}$$

(a) Non-cross resistant ↓ resistance problem
 eg, A (10^{-6}) + B (10^{-6}) = A + B (10^{-12})
(b) Dose (linear) = cell kill (exponential)
(c) Adjuvant chemotherapy, BMT in CR
(d) Clonal evolution → heterogeneity

Adjuvant chemotherapy

Adjuvant chemotherapy is for patients whose primary tumor has been controlled, but who are at high risk of having micrometastatic disease, and, therefore, late relapse and death. There is much experimental evidence that the treatment of microscopic forms of tumor is much more successful than the treatment of macroscopic overt cancer (Table 3). First, there is a lower tumor burden so that the kinetics are favorable. Second, the growth fraction, at least experimentally, for microscopic tumors is high and for big tumors, low. Most of our agents are relatively more effective against growing, ie, cycling cells. Cancers can outgrow their blood supply, so that for microscopic tumors the blood supply is putatively

Table 3 Adjuvant chemotherapy rationale.

	Metastatic lesions		
	Microscopic	Macroscopic	Comments
Tumor burden (no. cells)	$<10^8$	$>10^9 - 10^{10}$	Kinetics of tumor cell kill
Growth fraction	100%	<20%	Cell cycle-specific agents
Food supply	Intact	Hypovascular Angiogenesis	Drug distribution
Oxygen tension	Normal	Hypoxia	X ray, selected drugs require O_2
Mutation rates	↑	↑↑	Heterogeneity
Drug-resistant cells	↑	↑↑	Drug resistance

intact, whereas for bigger tumors, there is hypovascularity. This could adversely affect drug distribution. It could also affect oxygen concentration. Hypoxia is a feature of bigger tumors. Oxygen is essential for the therapeutic effects of X rays and certain chemotherapeutic agents; hypoxia is therefore a mechanism of resistance. Mutation rates are higher in larger and hypoxic tumors, and drug-resistant cells are therefore produced in greater quantities in these tumors. Therefore, if you want to cure a solid tumor, it should be treated when it is micrometastatic, ie, in the adjuvant setting.

Breast cancer

Breast cancer illustrates the use of adjuvant chemotherapy in the clinical setting. Breast cancer is the 2nd most common cause of death from cancer in women in the USA. A breast adjuvant CMF (cyclophosphamide, methotrexate, and fluorouracil [5FU]) trial was started in premenopausal patients by Bonadonna in 1972. Forty percent of patients in the control arm were surviving at 10 years. For the CMF arm the figure is 60%, a highly significant difference. The curves continue to separate and that separation has been maintained after 12 or 14 years (Fig 3).

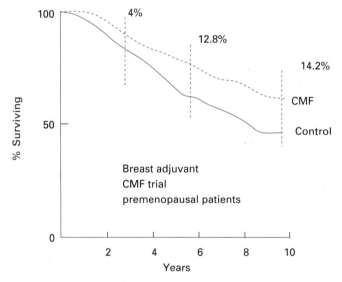

Fig 3 Survival in CMF trial premenopausal patients with breast cancer.

To determine the effects of adjuvant chemotherapy and tamoxifen, a metaanalysis of all published and extant studies was undertaken. For stage II patients there is a 15–20% reduction in the odds of mortality. Even for stage I patients with chemotherapy or tamoxifen, there is a 10–25% reduction in mortality [7].

35

What about the dose effect in adjuvant chemotherapy? Hyrniuk has defined "dose intensity" as integrating dose and schedule. It allows one to look at different programs, for example, CMF in breast cancer as a function of the actual dose delivered. His retrospective analysis of CMF-like programs shows that there is a steep dose-response curve with respect to the proportion of patients who are relapse free at 3 years (Fig 4) [8].

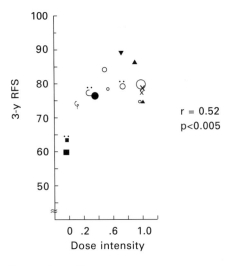

Fig 4 Breast cancer: adjuvant dose effect.

Since a retrospective study has limitations, the Cancer and Acute Leukemia Group B initiated a trial that has now accrued about 700 patients. In this trial, patients are randomly allocated to high-dose CAF (cyclophosphamide, doxorubicin, and 5FU) versus low-dose CAF. The difference in dose is 2-fold. The study is coded so we do not as yet know the results. This is an important study because it will determine prospectively the effect of dose, at least across a 2-fold range.

Neoadjuvant or induction chemotherapy

Neoadjuvant or induction chemotherapy is adjuvant chemotherapy taken to the front end of treatment protocols. Many patients, for example with head and neck cancer, have primary tumors that are large and invasive, such that the surgeon and/or the radiotherapist believe that they are incurable by local therapy. Under these circumstances, neoadjuvant chemotherapy is introduced to reduce the primary size and increase, hopefully, the chances of local control by surgery and radiotherapy. In addition, there is the importance of the earlier treatment of micrometastatic disease (Table 4) [9].

Table 4 Neoadjuvant (induction) chemotherapy.

- Strategy whose time has come
- Objectives
  - Down stage primary for subsequent S/R
  - Improve responsiveness of primary to R by ↑ blood supply and ↑ O_2
  - Earlier treatment of micrometastases (Goldie-Coldman)
  - In vivo assay of tumor responsiveness
  - Application:
    - Bladder, H&N, osteosarcoma, breast, childhood solid tumors, esophagus, cervical, regional lung
    - Problems, prospects: Biology of regressing primary, synchronous RT, better chemotherapy (S, S)

Goldie and Coldman and others, on the basis of theoretical studies and supportive data, have pointed out that micrometastases under certain circumstances can change from being drug sensitive to drug resistant in as little time as 2–4 months. Therefore, to wait to treat with adjuvant chemotherapy for as long as 3–4 months is potentially adverse. Neoadjuvant chemotherapy addresses micrometastatic disease early—a potentially important strategy.

We performed the following study in patients with head and neck cancer starting in 1980, so we have a long follow-up on approximately 114 patients (Fig 5). Eighty percent of the patients were stage IV, ie, advanced inoperable cancer. After 2 cycles of neoadjuvant or induction chemotherapy, the patients were restaged and received definitive surgery and/or radiotherapy, depending upon the primary tumor. The chemotherapy program involved a combination including cisplatin. We, and others, have found that even with the best combinations for patients who have had prior surgery and radiotherapy, only low complete response rates are produced (Table 5). However, if the same program is moved up front, substantially higher complete response rates are achieved.

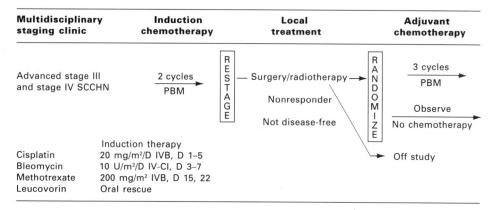

Fig 5 Neoadjuvant chemotherapy of head and neck cancer: protocol.

Table 5 Head and neck cancer response to neoadjuvant chemotherapy.

Treatment setting	Response rate (%)*	
	Total	Complete
Neoadjuvant	78–93	17–54
Post S/R	35–55	4–16

* Chemotherapy programs include: cisplatin +5FU
+Mtx, Bleo

Getting good responses in a local tumor is very important, but the durability of response and survival are critical. The patients who achieved complete response to chemotherapy had survival plateauing at 70–80% (Fig 6). In those who had a partial response or did not respond to chemotherapy, the survival was low. All neoadjuvant chemotherapy in head and neck cancer studies indicate the importance of complete response. This was not a controlled study, however, and it is possible that these patients differed in other ways. It is important to carry out prospective randomized studies to show that neoadjuvant chemotherapy does, in fact, benefit patients in terms of cure. Some 7 such studies have now been performed and most have been negative. They did not show that neoadjuvant chemotherapy improves survival. The problem with most of those studies, however, was that the complete response rate was low. If it is complete response only that affects survival, a complete response rate in excess of 20% would be needed even to see it in the context of a comparative study. We have therefore focused on increasing the complete response rate to above 20–25%. There are many approaches one can take to achieve this.

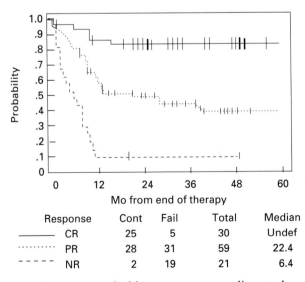

	Response	Cont	Fail	Total	Median
——	CR	25	5	30	Undef
········	PR	28	31	59	22.4
- - - -	NR	2	19	21	6.4

Fig 6 Head and neck cancer: survival by response to neoadjuvant chemotherapy.

Biochemical modulation

One approach toward increasing the complete response rate involves the addition of leucovorin to 5FU and cisplatin for neoadjuvant chemotherapy of head and neck cancer. This is referred to as modulation. 5FU is converted to FdUMP by several enzymatic steps, at which level it inhibits thymidylate synthase. The inhibition of thymidylate synthase is also very much dependent upon the binding of 5,10-methylene tetrahydrofolate to the enzyme. It can be shown, biochemically and in cells in culture, that the inhibition of thymidylate synthase by 5FU is greatly influenced by the quantity of methylene tetrahydrofolate bound to the enzyme and that can be increased in vitro and in vivo by the prodrug leucovorin. A number of randomized studies of metastatic colorectal cancer are currently in progress, wherein the control is 5FU and the treatment arm is 5FU plus leucovorin. The response rate has been substantially higher in the modulated 5FU arm, compared to 5FU only. Dreyfus and colleagues [10] at the Dana-Farber Cancer Institute have looked at this modulation in head and neck cancer and in 50 patients with stage IV inoperable disease found that the complete response rate was 60–70%. Of the patients who had clinically and radiographically a complete response, some 60–70% were, when rebiopsied or resected, pathologically free of tumor. If this is confirmed in other patients and if complete response affects survival, then this could translate into a meaningful increase in cure rate.

Dose and transplantation

Most of what I have reviewed above has involved relatively slight differences in dose, for example, a 2-fold difference. It is possible however, in the marrow transplantation situation, to increase doses of alkylating agents substantially (Table 6).

Table 6   Autologous bone marrow transplantation: dose effect.

Agent	Dose (mg/m^2)				Response (%)	
	Standard	Transplant	Ratio	Disease	Standard dose	Transplant dose
Carmustine	150	600–900	5	Melanoma	17	40–70 (10)
Melphalan	35	180–240	6	Melanoma	12	40–60 (15)
Melphalan	35	180–240	6	Colorectal	<10	40–50 (5)
CPA	600	5000–7000	10	—	—	—
Thiotepa	50	900–1150	20	Melanoma	10	50 (11)
TBI & CPA	—	—	>5	AML [A]	0	50 cure
CPA & busulfan	—	—	>5	AML [A]	0	50 cure

*CR + PR; ( ), CR. In patients with prior treatment.
[A] Also generally true for ALL, DHL, CML.

Total body irradiation (TBI) and cyclophosphamide used alone in the treatment of acute myelogenous leukemia (AML) in the past at standard dosages have not been effective. On the other hand, when used in the transplant setting, either autologuous or allogenic, a greater than 5-fold increase in dose can be delivered. Under these circumstances a 50% cure rate is achieved in patients with AML in complete remission. Santos substituted the alkylating agent busulfan for TBI and, again, a 50% cure rate in patients with AML was achieved. A similar picture is found with all the rapidly growing, hematologic neoplasms, such as non-Hodgkin's and Hodgkin's lymphoma, and acute lymphocytic leukemia. Can this be accomplished in patients with solid tumors? If one takes the individual alkylating agents and looks at the standard dose that can be delivered, and compares this to the maximum dose that can be delivered in the transplant situation, the increase ranges from 5- to 20-fold (Table 6). Researchers in preclinical in vivo systems have found that a 5-fold increase in dose is enough to produce a major increase in response. It is effective for relatively resistant, solid tumors which show a low, 10–15% response to the standard dose, but 40–70% for the transplant doses.

Alkylating agents are the main candidates for use in transplantation therapy, since it is for these agents that bone marrow toxicity is the dose-limiting factor. The alkylating agents are a heterogeneous group of compounds representing many classes and many individual agents (Table 7). The difficulty in the past was that, up to 10 years ago, alkylating agents were referred to as radiomimetic; they were thought to have a final common pathway similar to radiation and would be cross resistant among each other. That picture was changed by studies done by Schabel. When mouse leukemia L1210 in vivo was treated with cyclophosphamide, a 7 log kill was achieved. When the animals were treated in serial transplantation, a resistant line was produced. The expectation was that the line

Table 7 Alkylating agents: heterogeneity.

Chloroethyl amines
    HN_2, CPA (cyclophosphamide), PAM (phenylalanine mustard),
    chlorambucil, other
Platinum
    DDP, new analogues
Nitrosoureas
    BCNU, mCCNU, CCNU, streptozotocin
Epoxides
    DBD (dibromodulcitol, dibromomnnitol, galactitol)
Alkyl alkane sulfonates
    Busulfan, dimethylbusulfan
Aziridines
    TSPA, TEM
Monofunctional antitumor alkylating agents
    Procarbazine, DTIC

---

resistant to cyclophosphamide in vivo would be resistant to the other alkylating agents, ie, cross resistant. That turned out not to be the case. The same was true for melphalan, carmustine, and cisplatin. Schabel therefore reversed the prevailing dogma by showing that alkylating agents were mostly not cross resistant with each other. So alkylating agents could be used in combination, particularly in the transplant arena, and that was the basis of our solid tumor autologuous marrow program.

Obviously what exists experimentally may not be true of human tumor cells. Because of this, we began to look at the process of drug resistance in human tumor cell lines (Fig 7). For the antimetabolites generally, illustrated for methotrexate here, one can produce very high levels of resistance [11]. For the nonalkylating agents as a generalization, one can also produce in vitro high levels of resistance. This is not so for the alkylating agents. With selection pressure over several months, the concentration that can be delivered is increased, after which, if the concentration is increased further, all the cells die. When these cells were cloned we found that there was resistance of 3- to 12-fold, but never more than that. So the alkylating agents are unique among chemotherapeutic agents in that it is difficult for cells to develop high levels of resistance. That in itself is an important quality for any agent [12].

Such a characteristic has implications for dose. If one can deliver a high dose, such as in the transplantation arena, that dose theoretically could provide a concentration to which cells could not be or become resistant. The alkylating agents in this sense will closely resemble radiation, with which it has been extremely difficult in vitro or in vivo to produce significant levels of resistance.

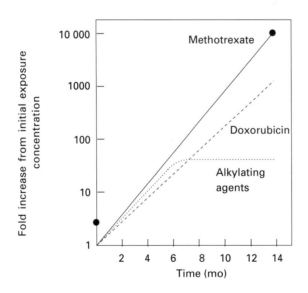

Fig 7 Schema of the development of resistance using selection pressure.

We found when we looked for cross resistance among the cell lines that Schabel was generally correct, ie, there was either no cross resistance or low levels of cross resistance. One of the implications of lack of cross resistance is of course the potential for the use of alkylating agents in combination. Schabel realized this and showed that a number of combinations of alkylating agents were synergistic in experimental systems. Teicher looked at thiotepa plus cyclophosphamide in a human breast cancer cell line, MCF7, which is a commonly used model. She found that for cyclophosphamide, low doses of thiotepa were synergistic, a synergism that has been important for us because we have used this combination in our clinical studies (Fig 8).

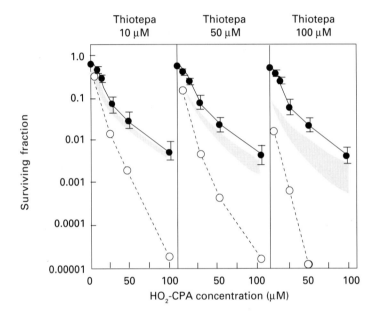

Fig 8 Thiotepa and cyclophosphamide combination against human breast cancer: MCF7 in vitro.

Clinical studies

The intitial program for our clinical protocol, STAMP (Solid Tumor Autologous Marrow Program) started 6–7 years ago and involves cyclophosphamide, cisplatin, and carmustine. We took agents, all of which were available in the clinic, that had activity in solid tumors and that represented different classes of alkylating agents. These were also, at least in our preclinical experience, agents which were not cross resistant with each other.

In a phase I study we worked up to transplantation doses. The marrow was harvested, the intensive chemotherapy delivered, the autologuous marrow returned, and essentially all patients reconstituted. There is a 3–4 week period during which the patient must be isolated, protected, and treated expectantly and supportively. Unfortunately, there was toxicity and a 15% mortality in patients with advanced refractory solid tumors. In terms of response rate, our experience was gratifying, in that the overall partial and complete response rate was 80% (Table 8). Peters has continued to use that program with success in patients with breast cancer. The key factor is whether it is going to be possible to translate those responses into long-term, tumor-free survival. We do not yet know the answer to that [13].

Table 8 Response to STAMP1.

Disease	No.	UE	NR	PR	CR	%RR/E
Breast	19	3	1	9	6	94
Melanoma	20	2	6	11	1	67
Sarcoma	8	2	0	5	1	100
Lung (NSC)	4	2	0	2	0	100
Colon	2	0	2	0	0	0
Lymphoma	3	0	0	2	1	100
Ovarian	2	0	0	2	0	100
Testis	1	1	0	0	0	–
Lung (small cell)	1	1	0	0	0	–
Total	61	10	9	34	9	

UE, unevaluable (<4 weeks observation);
NR, no response (<50% response);
PR, partial response (50–99% reponse);
CR, complete response (100% response);
RR, response rate (%PR + CR);
E, evaluable patients.

Dr Antman and her colleagues have done a series of phase I studies. Herzig found that a marked increase in dose of thiotepa could be delivered in the context of transplantation. Thiotepa is non-cross-resistant with cyclophosphamide, it is synergistic with cyclophosphamide, and we therefore carried out a phase I study of the combination of cyclophosphamide and thiotepa. We did not favor cisplatin as an agent for transplantation because of dose-limiting toxicity to the kidney and the nervous system. This is obviously not something that would be avoided by bone marrow transplantation. On the other hand, the analogue carboplatin is therapeutically generally the equivalent to cisplatin. However, for carboplatin dose-limiting toxicity is related to its bone marrow effects. Shea demonstrated that carboplatin in the context of bone marrow transplantation could be increased by 6–8 times the standard dose. Thus, carboplatin appeared to be the better agent for use in transplantation. We therefore added carboplatin to these 2 agents in a phase I study and we are now performing a phase II study in patients with breast cancer with cyclophosphamide, thiotepa, and carboplatin (CTC) [14].

Our study protocol enters patients with stage IV metastatic breast cancer, who have not received prior chemotherapy. In order to minimize the tumor burden and demonstrate responsiveness to chemotherapy, the patients are initially treated with AMF, that is a doxorubicin-based combination. This is, therefore, induction chemotherapy. Those 80% of patients who respond go on to intensification with the STAMP protocol, involving CTC. This study now has accrued 25 patients.

Data collected by Dr Antman indicate the importance of combination chemotherapy and prior treatment to responsiveness to transplantation in patients with breast cancer. She showed that the complete response rate was only 5% for single agents employed in refractory patients. It rose to a 25% complete response rate when combinations were used in refractory patients. It was almost 50% when combinations were used in patients with no prior chemotherapy, and some 75% when combinations were employed in patients who were responding to prior induction therapy. This demonstrated that combinations are important and prior treatment is adverse [15].

We have seen that for acute lymphocytic leukemia and Hodgkin's disease, the first event leading ultimately to curative impact is achievement of a high complete response rate. This, at least, appears to have happened with the STAMP-like programs. Whether this can be translated into long-term disease-free survival and cure remains to be seen. One model that is being used by Peters at Duke University is in patients with stage II disease, that is, in patients with a lower tumor burden, but patients at substantial risk of fatality from their disease in that they have 10 or more positive lymph nodes. These patients have their primary tumor controlled and then go through a similar regimen to that described above for patients with stage IV disease [16].

Future directions

Some of the approaches designed to improve the transplantation chemotherapy regimen involve finding better alkylating agents, better schedules, and improved doses which we are pursuing in ongoing studies. Another approach has been thrown into relief by studies of the mechanism of resistance to alkylating agents (Table 9). It appears that there are a variety of mechanisms of resistance, including membrane transport, glutathione, glutathione transferase, and DNA damage and repair. All of these have been found to explain resistance and usually, resistance is multifactorial. If that is correct and one wants to modulate these mechanisms to sensitivity, it makes sense to employ a combination of modulation agents.

Such modulation can be approached in different ways. One can lower reduced glutathione (GSH), which is a scavenger for alkylating agents, by using an inhibitor of GSH synthesis. One can lower certain isozymes of glutathione transferase with compounds such as ethacrynic acid. The blood substitute Fluosol can deliver oxygen into the center of tumors and thereby increase DNA

Table 9 Alkylating agent resistance: heterogeneity.

Membrane transport
- choline - HN^2*
- leucine amino acid - PAM*
- ? cisplatin
Intracellular binding, metabolism
- ↑GSH, PAM, cisplatin, other
- ↑GT, cisplatin
- ↑protein - SH (metallothionein), chlorambucil, cisplatin
- ↑aldehyde oxidase, CPA*
Increase DNA repair
- ↑0^6 methyl transferase, carmustine*
- Other (alkaline elution), PAM
Efflux
- ? MDR

*Specific for selecting agent.

damage through reducing hypoxic levels. At the level of DNA repair, it has been possible using topoisomerase II inhibitors and materials that shorten the G2 period of the cell cycle, thereby decreasing DNA repair. These approaches increase the effectiveness of alkylating agents in experimental systems and are in phase I clinical trials being conducted currently.

References

1. Frei E III. Curative cancer chemotherapy. Cancer Res 1985;45:6523–37.
2. Frei E III, Canellos GP. Dose: a critical factor in cancer chemotherapy. Am J Med 1980;69:585–94.
3. Pinkel D, Hernandez K, Borella L, et al. Drug dosage and remission duration in childhood lymphocytic leukemia. Cancer 1971;37:247–56.
4. Frei E III. Pathobiology of cancer. In: Scientific American Medicine, vol 2.
5. Frei E III, DeVita VT, Moxley JH III, Carbone PP. Approaches to improving the chemotherapy of Hodgkin's disease. Cancer Res 1966;26:1284–9.
6. DeVita VT, Serpick A, Carbone PP. Combination chemotherapy in the treatment of advanced Hodgkin's disease. Ann Intern Med 1970;73:881.
7. Early Breast Cancer Trialists' Collaborative Group. Effects of early adjuvant tamoxifen and of cytotoxic therapy on mortality in early breast cancer. N Engl J Med 1988;319: 1681–92.
8. Hryniuk W, Bonadonna G, Valagussa P. The effect of dose intensity in adjuvant chemotherapy. In: Salmon SE, ed. Adjuvant therapy of cancer V. Orlando, FL: Grune & Stratton; 1987:13–23.
9. Clark JR, Fallon BG, Frei E III. Induction chemotherapy as initial treatment for advanced head and neck cancer: a model for the multidisciplinary treatment of solid tumors. In: DeVita VT, Jr, Hellman SK, Rosenberg SA, eds. Important advances in oncology 1987. Philadelphia: JB Lippincott; 1987:221–35.

10. Dreyfuss A, Clark JR, Wright JE, et al. Continuous infusion high-dose leucovorin with 5-fluorouracil and cisplatin for untreated stage IV carcinoma of the head and neck. Ann Intern Med 1990;112:167–72.
11. Frei E III, Cucchi CA, Rosowsky A, et al. Alkylating agent resistance: in vitro studies with human cell lines. Proc Natl Acad Sci USA 1985;82:2158–62.
12. Frei E III, Teicher BA, Holden SA, et al. Preclinical studies and clinical correlation of the effect of alkylating dose. Cancer Res 1988;48:6417–23.
13. Antman K, Peters WP, Eder JP, et al. Treatment of 58 patients on a phase I and II protocol using a high-dose combination alkylating agent preparative regimen with autologous bone marrow support. In: Fortner JG, Rhoads JE, eds. Accomplishments in cancer research. Philadelphia: JB Lippincott; 1985:152–65.
14. Peters WP, Eder JP, Henner WD, et al. Novel toxicities associated with high dose combination alkylating agents and autologous bone marrow support. In: Dicke K, Spitzer G, Zander AR, eds. Autologous bone marrow transplantation: proceedings of the 1st international symposium. Houston: University of Texas M.D. Anderson Hospital and Tumor Institute; 1985:231–5.
15. Antman K. Personal communication.
16. Peters W. Personal communication.

Discussion

Chairperson: **Kiyoji Kimura**

Dr Makoto Ogawa (Cancer Chemotherapy Center, Japanese Foundation for Cancer Research, Tokyo): I would like to ask 2 questions. One is related to neoadjuvant chemotherapy for head and neck tumors. What do you consider to be the optimal number of cycles of chemotherapy?

Dr Frei: Our rule is that for a patient who achieves a complete remission by 2 cycles, further cycles are unnecessary, so we go on to local treatment. For patients who achieve a partial response after 2 courses of therapy, and particularly for those who exhibit evidence of continuing tumor regression, we add a 3rd course. If patients do not respond by 2 courses of chemotherapy, they are not destined to respond to further treatment with the same chemotherapy. That has been our strategy, but it needs to be reexamined in the light of different neoadjuvant combinations.

Dr Ogawa: So do you think 2 cycles are enough to get complete remission?

Dr Frei: I should qualify this by saying that with our new program that involves leucovorin, we have decided to go to 3 cycles almost as a routine, because again, partial responders, who are the majority of patients, at least they have been in the past, are the ones most likely to benefit from a 3rd course, so whether it is 2 or 3, I am not sure. Maybe it is more than 3 for certain types of programs.

Dr Ogawa: My 2nd question is related to the patient receiving high-dose chemotherapy with autologous bone marrow transplantation. For the patient who obtains a complete remission with high-dose chemotherapy, do you offer any additional chemotherapy, that is, maintenance, or consolidation therapy?

Dr Frei: We do not offer any additional chemotherapy, as long as patients are in complete remission, but we do have another element in our strategy, that is a 3rd element, which I did not discuss in my presentation. It turns out that for cancer generally—it was first observed for Hodgkin's disease, but it is largely

47

true for all solid tumors—that if you give patients with metastatic disease systemic treatment, the site of relapse is very predictable; it is where they had pretreatment bulk tumor. Because of that, patients in complete remission are at high risk of relapsing in those areas, presumably because they have persisting microscopic disease and because of this, our strategy has been, where possible, to identify such areas and to irradiate such areas locally after they are in complete remission from chemotherapy.

Dr Hisashi Majima (Ichijokai Hospital, Ichikawa):   I would like to ask an extension of Dr Ogawa's question. In head and neck cancer you said you give 2 courses of chemotherapy. If this is good enough for surgical removal, then do you send the patient to the surgical department or do you give more courses until the patient reaches CR? Do you give postoperative chemo- or radiotherapy?

Dr Frei: The question really is the importance of using chemotherapy postoperatively as well as preoperatively.

Dr Majima: Do you press on to the endpoint with neoadjuvant chemotherapy for a partial response, good enough for surgical removal?

Dr Frei: That is a complicated, but very important question, which is being addressed in the context of clinical trials. One problem is that patients with head and neck cancer, after 2 or 3 courses before surgery and then surgery and/or radiotherapy, are often not good candidates for further chemotherapy, because, in a sense, they have had enough. So it is not an easy question to answer. One could use adjuvant chemotherapy and this has been done with primary treatment of head and neck cancer followed by chemotherapy. We still think that it is important to look at the biology of solid tumor regression with chemotherapy because there are a lot of things that happen that we do not understand. We expect that the blood supply would become relatively greater, that hypoxia would become less. We are not sure whether the tumor would decrease in size or stay the same, decrease in density, and soften. All of these possibilities have major implications for what should be the nature of follow-up local treatment and whether or not they need further chemotherapy. If the blood supply is improved, if hypoxia is controlled, that ought to make radiotherapy better. If the tumor shrinks and the invasive edges of the tumor retreat, that ought to make surgery better. There is some evidence that I think is still controversial, but it is very interesting, that patients who have a very good response, for example, a complete response to chemotherapy, may not require radical surgery, and may do just as well with radiotherapy. There may be an ascendancy of radiotherapy use as a result of neoadjuvant chemotherapy, but as yet we have not come to any conclusion about this.

Dr Nagahiro Saijo (National Cancer Center, Tokyo): You stressed that a complete response is required for the improvement of survival in patients who receive neoadjuvant chemotherapy. I think that there are several neoadjuvant trials in stage IIIA non-small cell lung cancer which have shown a response rate of about 60–70%. However, the CR rate is probably less than 10%. Do you think that this kind of strategy is reasonable or should we change the target of patients, especially those in stage I or II?

Dr Frei: Neoadjuvant chemotherapy is being studied, not only in head and neck cancer, but in breast cancer, in non-small cell lung cancer, in bladder cancer very importantly, in osteogenic sarcoma, so as a strategy it is something that is very much with us and again is under study. In the instance you cite, that is patients with non-small cell lung cancer, that is the big question, in a sense, that is a major cause of death from cancer, and neoadjuvant chemotherapy has been looked at in patients with so-called regional stage IIIA disease particularly (regional disease means a primary as well as involvement of the mediastinum), or A and B disease, which depends on the extent of involvement of the mediastinum. There have been 5 or 6 comparative studies of neoadjuvant chemotherapy followed by radiotherapy versus radiotherapy alone in stage III non-small cell lung cancers. Most of them showed no difference in terms of survival. In the CALGB study, there was a highly significant difference in favor of the neoadjuvant chemotherapy arm, that is vinblastine plus cisplatin. The 2 curves that parted about 2-fold, with about a 14–15 month median survival for the treated arm and 7–8 months for the control arm, and at 2 years, with a plateau, it was about 25% for the treated arm and about 8% or 10% for the control arm. That is not a big difference, but the difference was significant in the context of about 200 patients, so highly significant that the monitoring committee terminated the study. Why was that study positive, and the other similar studies negative? We are not sure, but I would proffer this explanation and that is that in the CALGB study, only patients with good performance status, ie, 1 or 0, were entered, whereas in the other studies, patients with status 2 or 3 were allowed as well. I think whenever you are looking for a difference in a sensitive situation and you dilute the experience with patients who are generally less responsive, as poor performance status patients are, you diminish the possibility of seeing a difference. That is *an* explanation, but whether it is *the* explanation, I am not sure. However, our study does stand as a positive study.

Dr Saijo: I would like to ask why you believe that there is no cross resistance between alkylating agents. The reason why I ask this question is as follows: we have established 5 cisplatin-resistant lines; these cell lines are completely cross resistant with alkylating agents. If we check several factors of drug resistance, however, drug uptake is only about 2- or 3-fold different and the glutathione level is also only 2- or 3-fold different in one cell line. However, in other cell lines, drug uptake is 5- or 8-fold different, so I think with alkylating agents the mechanism for each drug-resistant cell line is different from cell to cell. What is your opinion on this?

Dr Frei: I know your studies and they are elegant and I certainly did not mean to imply that there was no cross resistance at all among the alkylating agents. In fact, there are frequently low levels of cross resistance and sometimes relatively high levels of cross resistance in our experience. I think the reason for that is again multifactorial; there are so many ways in which drugs can become resistant to alkylating agents, that they often do it in a multifactorial fashion and that probably teleologically and in an evolutionary way makes sense as well. I think the expectation is that resistance is multifactorial. It does mean that we need multiple modulating approaches and that low levels of cross resistance may relate to one of several mechanisms of resistance.

Dr Shigeru Tsukagoshi (Cancer Chemotherapy Center, Japanese Foundation for Cancer Research, Tokyo):   You mentioned heterogeneity of the tumor cells to drug sensitivity, but in the clinical situation, do you think that similar heterogeneity is maintained after relapse?

Dr Frei: We like to think of minimal disease at the front end as comparable to minimal disease that we induce after treatment, for instance after debulking in patients with ovarian cancer, but it is not the same at all. Goldie has pointed out that resistance is related to the length of the mitotic history as much as anything else, and cells that have become minimal and then persisted for a period of time have been in existence mitotically for a much longer period than new disease. So I would expect that for a given amount of disease, patients who have had relapses would be intrinsically more likely to have drug resistance than earlier patients. I think clinical and laboratory experience as well bears that out pretty well.

Dr Kiyoji Kimura (National Nagoya Hospital and Nagoya Memorial Hospital, Nagoya):   What do you think about the collateral sensitivity that might be induced by the alternative use of anticancer agents?

Dr Frei: A very important question. There are certainly a number of circumstances where the production of resistance to one drug increases the sensitivity to other drugs. That was first shown for 6-mercaptopurine resistance by Dr Lloyd Law, because 6-mercaptopurine resistance related to loss of the salvage pathways for purines, and therefore the cells, was more sensitive to methotrexate, which destroyed de novo synthesis of purine. So that was the expectation and it was true; the biochemical evidence was conclusive. There is some evidence that alkylating agent-resistant cells are more sensitive to anthracyclines and maybe also to vinca alkaloids. We are not quite sure why that is true. It may relate to topoisomerase II. While cross resistance among alkylating agents exists particularly at low levels and is of concern in terms of their use in combination, is important to recognize that multidrug resistance research now indicates that seemingly unrelated drugs, such as vincristine, vinblastine, doxorubicin, and dactinomycin, can often be cross resistant with each other and yet we use those commonly in combination in the clinic. So the laboratory and the clinic have to come together on these important issues.

Head and neck cancer

The role of induction chemotherapy in advanced head and neck cancer

Waun Ki Hong

The University of Texas M.D. Anderson Cancer Center, Houston, Texas

Introduction

Although induction chemotherapy has been used in the USA since 1978, it is still considered to be investigational and experimental. In this review, I will focus on the role of induction chemotherapy for organ preservation in head and neck cancer. I believe this is a very exciting area and has the potential to make an impact as a new treatment modality in head and neck cancer [1,2].

As is well known, the early stages of head and neck cancer can be treated by surgical excision and/or radiotherapy (XRT). This produces an excellent cure rate without compromising any organ function. However, the therapeutic problem remains for head and neck cancer patients in advanced stages III and IV. The prognosis for stages III and IV is extremely poor, despite the humiliating and debilitating treatment the patient may have to undergo. Some patients who are fortunate enough to survive their cancer have to face a lifetime of significant morbidity, due to cosmetic and functional debilities from surgical treatment. Clearly, new approaches for improvement in both patient survival and quality of life need to be explored. This then raises the question: what is the role of induction chemotherapy in the treatment of head and neck cancer? Unfortunately, previous randomized trials of induction chemotherapy failed to show any improvement in survival. However, improvements in quality of life need to be addressed as well as survival rates. It is important, therefore, to look at whether induction chemotherapy fulfills any other role, such as organ and function preservation, thus improving the patient's quality of life. To address this specific issue, I will first review several induction chemotherapy studies that have supported the concept of organ function preservation. Second, I will consider laryngeal cancer as an outstanding model for testing that hypothesis. Finally, I will briefly discuss some other head and neck sites for organ function preservation and future directions for research.

Induction chemotherapy for organ preservation

Since conventional chemotherapy for salvaging recurrent head and neck cancer patients has yielded such poor results, other chemotherapy protocols have been tried. Induction chemotherapy has been incorporated in a neoadjuvant setting prior to surgery and/or radiation therapy and also given in a sequential or a simultaneous fashion with XRT. Some patients with paranasal sinus cancer have been treated with intraarterial chemotherapy, followed by surgery and XRT.

The major rationale for using induction chemotherapy is to obtain better control. Induction chemotherapy prior to surgery and/or radiation treatment would theoretically eliminate the pharmacological sanctuary. Patients receiving such induction chemotherapy would have better performance and nutritional status, both of which are very important prognostic factors for response to chemotherapy in most tumors. The chemotherapy would also induce cytoreduction and therefore enhance local regional control. This strategy may also be important in eliminating subclinical micrometastases in patients with locally advanced cancer. Some concerns have been expressed, however, mainly by surgeons and radiotherapists. Induction chemotherapy can increase local toxicity from XRT. It can also cause other problems, such as delayed surgery, inadequate identification of negative margins at the time of surgery, and increased postoperative complications. Chemotherapy toxicity can cause immunosuppression with morbidity and, rarely, mortality.

Table 1 shows the induction regimens administered during the past 10 years in the USA. The combination induction regimen appears to be superior to the single agent in terms of complete response rate, with response rates of 60–90% being achieved (Table 1). So far, the combination cisplatin and fluorouracil (5FU) regimen from Wayne State University (Detroit) appears to be the most effective induction regimen, with a complete response rate of over 30% in advanced head and neck cancer [3–6]. Many other cisplatin-containing regimens have been administered; as they do not seem superior to the cisplatin/5FU regimen, overall response rates have remained low.

As radiotherapy alone achieves poor results in patients with advanced inoperable head and neck cancer, chemotherapy followed by XRT has been investi-

Table 1 Induction chemotherapy regimens.

Chemotherapy regimen	No. of patients	Overall RR (CR + PR)
Single agent (MTX, DDP, or bleomycin)	188	45% (2 + 43)
Cisplatin + bleomycin	467	48% (7 + 41)
Cisplatin + bleomycin + MTX	323	74% (16 + 58)
Cisplatin + bleomycin + vinca alkaloid	474	69% (20 + 49)
Cisplatin + 5FU	461	86% (35 + 51)

MTX, methotrexate; DDP, cisplatin.

gated. This sequential strategy for decreasing tumor bulk thereby decreases the number of hypoxic cells. The chemotherapeutic agent could also function as a radiosensitizer; however, several randomized studies have shown no survival benefit. Sequential chemotherapy and XRT appear to induce a higher local control rate than XRT alone [2,6].

In terms of defining the role of induction chemotherapy in organ preservation, the most innovative study was conducted by Jacobs at Stanford University, who attempted to determine whether induction chemotherapy could eliminate radical surgery, if the patient showed complete response to chemotherapy [7]. Patients with resectable stages III and IV head and neck cancer were treated with an induction regimen using platinum/5FU for 3 cycles. Complete responders then had a biopsy. If the biopsy was negative, the patient then received radiation instead of surgery. Patients who showed a persistent tumor on biopsy specimens, and patients who did not show any or only a partial response to induction chemotherapy received standard treatment, ie, surgery and radiation. Although the numbers were small, the Jacobs study strongly suggested that in patients with resectable stages III and IV cancer who achieve a pathologic complete remission with induction chemotherapy, it is feasible to eliminate radical surgery. Instead, patients can be treated with primary XRT without compromising survival (Table 2). Furthermore, several studies by other investigators have shown that the response to induction chemotherapy also predicts further response to radiation treatment and, conversely, chemotherapy nonresponders have a poor response to radiation therapy (Table 3).

Data from many large trials of induction chemotherapy have also been analyzed for prognostic factors for response to chemotherapy. So far, TN stage and

Table 2 Results with induction CT as a substitute for radical surgery. Reprinted, with permission, from Jacobs et al [7].

	% 2-y DFS	2-y Overall survival
Entire group (n=30)	52	53
CR+ XRT (n=10)	60	70

Table 3 Tumor response to XRT followng induction chemotherapy.

Investigator(s)	Ref no.	Responders (%)	Nonresponders (%)
Glick, 1980	8	64	10
Hill & Price, 1988	9	72	45
Ensley et al, 1984	10	52	6
Hong et al, 1985	11	71	17

type of induction chemotherapy regimen have proved to be the most important prognostic factors for response to chemotherapy [7,8]. Many investigators have demonstrated superior survival in complete responders to induction chemotherapy, compared to partial responders and nonresponders, although this may just reflect identification of the prognostically favorable group. Response to induction chemotherapy, particularly complete response, is of major importance because of the excellent correlation between histologic complete response and clinical complete response.

Many exciting, nonrandomized studies are being conducted and several randomized trials have also been reported in the literature, with survival as the endpoint. Unfortunately, all the randomized studies failed to show any survival benefit (Table 4). The question now is, "What should we do next?" Should we abandon the use of induction chemotherapy because it has no survival benefit in head and neck cancer patients?

Table 4 Randomized trials of induction chemotherapy.

Investigator	Ref no.	Regimen	No. of patients	% CR + PR	Overall survival benefit
Stell, 1983	15	Price-Hill	86	Not mentioned	None
Schuller, 1984	13	DDP + Bleo + VCR	146	20 + 25	None
Kun, 1986	16	BLEO + CMF	83	5 + 63	None
Martin, 1986	17	DDP + BLEO	60	7 + 57	None
Toohill, 1987	14	DDP + 5 FU	60	19 + 67	None
NCI contract, 1987	12	DDP + BLEO	462	3 + 34	None

DDP, cisplatin; Bleo, bleomycin; VCR, vincristine; MTX, methotrexate; LV, leucovorin; CMF, cyclophosphamide + MTX + 5FU.

A critical look at the randomized studies is required. We then find that they all used a single agent or an ineffective regimen, or an effective regimen but at a suboptimal dose or with an inconsistent schedule. Therefore, low complete response rates were obtained. Also, one UK study appeared to show attenuation of the radiation dose in the chemotherapy group, so they did not receive the standard dose of radiation treatment [15]. The very small sample size and inadequate follow-up in this trial also make it difficult to draw any meaningful conclusions.

To summarize, a great deal of positive knowledge has been gained since induction chemotherapy was first introduced more than a decade ago. It is a feasible treatment, it does not increase surgical or XRT complications, the response rate correlates with the tumor burden, response to chemotherapy is predictive for further response to radiation treatment, a high complete response can be obtained with the effective regimen, and the pathologic complete response is correlated with the clinical complete response in about one half of the patients [18]. Patients who achieve a complete response do have improved survival. Furthermore, radical surgery may be omitted in patients who achieve complete pathologic remission. However, some negative points regarding induction chemotherapy were also identified: chemotherapy prolongs the already lengthy treatment course, treatment is expensive, and the patient may refuse to undergo local therapy after excellent response to initial chemotherapy. The Wayne State University group has reported up to a 40% refusal rate for the definitive treatment and the later palliative treatment period with chemotherapy may be compromised. Again, randomized studies have shown that there is no survival benefit. The obvious question is: how can we take advantage of the positive aspects of induction chemotherapy obtained from previous trials of the organ preservation approach in head and neck cancer? Laryngeal cancer is an excellent model for testing the organ preservation hypothesis.

Laryngeal cancer as a model for organ preservation

The standard treatment for operable stages III and IV laryngeal cancer in the USA is total laryngectomy and postoperative XRT. Unfortunately, the patients lose their natural speech as a consequence of the laryngectomy. Of major concern are the functional, psychological, and cosmetic deformities resulting from the laryngectomy. The standard treatment for a small lesion of the larynx, such as a T1 lesion, is either radiation or surgery. Even with a T2 lesion of the larynx, approximately 3 out of 5 patients can be cured with radiation treatment. Patients with advanced stages T3 and T4 lesions with nodular disease, however, are given standard treatment, ie, surgery and radiation. The problems associated with the standard treatment in this case are not only poor survival, but that patients also lose the larynx. Upfront surgery, ie, laryngectomy, and radiation treatment, can improve some survival at the expense of impaired speech. However, XRT upfront may save the larynx, but at the price of a decreased chance of survival (Table 5) [19–21].

Table 5 Results of alternative treatment in advanced laryngeal cancer. Reprinted, with permission, from McNeil BJ et al [21].

	3-y survival (%)	
	Stage III	Stage IV
Primary laryngectomy	40 – 50	30 – 40
XRT	20 – 30	<20
XRT and salvage surgery	30 – 40	20 – 30
Laryngectomy and XRT	40 – 60	30 – 50
Induction CT and XRT		
with salvage surgery	?	?

Because XRT alone and XRT with surgical laryngectomy achieve very poor outcomes in advanced laryngeal cancer, several investigators in the USA have studied the approach using induction chemotherapy followed by radiation therapy, in an attempt to preserve the larynx for patients who would otherwise have required a laryngectomy. Table 6 shows several nonrandomized studies that were carried out using sequential chemotherapy and radiation therapy that clearly

Table 6 Laryngeal preservation with CT and XRT in patients in whom total laryngectomy would have been done initially.

Investigator	Ref no.	No. of patients	CR after CT	CR after CT	Comments
Hong	11	20	3 (15%)	16 (80%)	Med. surv. 23 mo
Karp	22	34	8 (24%)	19 (56%)	Med. surv. 23 mo
Haines	23	24	10 (42%)	17 (71%)	57% NED at median F/U 19 mo
Hill	9	73	–	59 (81%)	Median surv. 53 mo

show promising results. At least in the majority of patients, the larynx was initially preserved without compromising survival.

VA Laryngeal Cancer Study

The strategy of using induction chemotherapy and XRT in advanced laryngeal cancer is currently under investigation by the VA Laryngeal Study Group [24], which consists of 12 VA hospitals in the USA. The rationale behind this study was based on data from pilot studies that showed that such a strategy might be feasible and well tolerated; induction chemotherapy induced a high complete response rate and response to chemotherapy predicted response to radiation therapy, and the partial responses were converted to complete responses with radiation treatment. We know that XRT is very effective in controlling small-sized tumors. The bottom line is that we would also like to preserve the human larynx. To be eligible for the VA study, patients must have operable stages III/IV squamous cell carcinoma of the larynx, excluding T1N1. The patients must also have a good perfomance status (>50 on the Karnofsky scale) and normal renal and hematologic functions.

We designed a randomized study to determine whether induction chemotherapy followed by radiation therapy is an alternative to, or improvement on, the standard treatment of surgery and postoperative XRT. In the experimental arm, the patient receives induction chemotherapy for 2 cycles. This is important. For induction chemotherapy we give cisplatin and 5FU, and patients who show a response after 2 cycles receive an additional cycle of chemotherapy. Patients who do not show any response after 2 cycles are immediately given standard treatment, ie, surgery and radiation. In patients who receive the 3rd cycle of chemotherapy, the response is assessed by direct endoscopy, in most patients, and histologic evaluation is also performed. Patients then receive the standard dose of radiation treatment, 6600–7600 rad. Twelve weeks after radiation treatment they are assessed again and patients who show no evidence of disease are followed. Any patient who shows persistent residual disease is biopsied and undergoes surgical laryngectomy. So we perform 2 different types of salvage laryngectomy: before and after radiation (Figure).

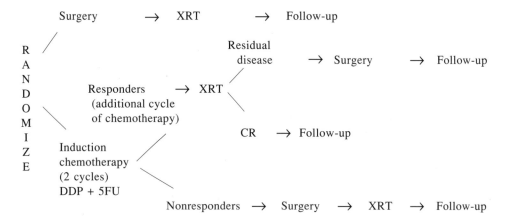

Figure Veterans Administration Cooperative Study Program Trial (VACSP). DDP, cisplatin. DDP, 100 mg/m^2 iv; 5FU, 1000 mg/m^2 for 5 days, continuous infusion.

The VA study was started in January 1985 and 332 patients had been randomized by the end of March 1989. One hundred and sixty-six patients received surgery and radiation treatment, and another 166 received induction chemotherapy and radiation treatment. The interim survival data of VACSP were presented in May 1989 at the American Society of Clinical Oncology meeting in San Francisco [24]. The patient characteristics are shown in Table 8. There were no significant differences between the groups in terms of factors considered to influence prognosis, such as patients' performance status, primary tumor site, or tumor stage. The 2 groups were well balanced.

Tumor response was assessed after the 2nd and 3rd cycles of chemotherapy. After the 2nd cycle, 147 patients were evaluable for tumor response: 24% achieved a clinical complete response and 60% obtained a partial response. Nonresponders immediately underwent salvage laryngectomy according to the protocol. One hundred and twenty-four patients were eligible to receive a 3rd cycle of treatment and 108 patients were evaluable for response. Of the 108, 40%

obtained a complete response and 56% a partial response. Four patients were considered to be nonresponders because of disease progression during the 3rd cycle of chemotherapy. The 97 patients who completed the 3rd cycle of chemotherapy were also biopsied superficially at the primary site for histologic evaluation. On direct endoscopy, the biopsy was negative in 63% of the patients.

Chemotherapy toxicity was also analyzed in 108 patients. The major side effects were from gastrointestinal tract toxicity, primarily nausea, vomiting, and diarrhea. Other toxicity was mainly very mild or moderate neutropenia and mild renal toxicity. However, 11 patients developed a grade II or III toxicity and 1 patient died of chemotherapy-related complications.

The relapse-free interval was calculated from randomization to documented recurrent disease using the Kaplan-Meier method. The relapse-free intervals showed no significant difference at a median follow-up of 23 months. The estimated 2-year relapse-free survival was 67% in the surgical group, compared with 63% in the chemotherapy group (Table 5).

The survival curve includes all patients entered into this trial. Survival was calculated from randomization to the last follow-up visit. The patient survival curves again show no difference at a median follow-up of 23 months. The estimated 2-year survival rate of each treatment group was identical at 66%. It is interesting to note the patterns of relapse in both the surgical group and the chemotherapy group. The total relapse rate was 32% in the surgical group compared with 37% in the chemotherapy group. In the chemotherapy group, the majority of the initial failures were the local and the regional tumors, as might be expected. The finding of a smaller proportion of distant metastases in the chemotherapy group was interesting; the pattern of failure was quite different in the surgical group, which had more distant metastases. Twenty-six patients developed distant metastases in the surgical group compared to only 10 patients in the group that received chemotherapy and radiation. There was also a very low relapse rate in local and regional sites in the surgical group. These findings strongly suggest that an improved technique must be devised to improve local tumor control when combination chemotherapy and radiation therapy are given for advanced laryngeal cancer.

Twenty-nine patients in the chemotherapy group and 15 in the surgical group are receiving active treatment. Of the 128 patients who have completed treatment, 80 are alive and 54 of them (68%) are alive with an intact larynx. In the surgical group, only 7 out of 103 patients (7%) are alive with an intact larynx, which, it should be emphasized, is only a partial larynx. Therefore, we can conclude that the fairly high clinical and histologic response rates and acceptable toxicity indicate the feasibility of this approach for head and neck cancer, especially advanced laryngeal cancer. This approach has demonstrated so far that the human larynx can be initially preserved in most patients, as 54 of 128 patients (42%) who completed the treatment are still alive with an intact larynx after a median follow-up of about 31 months. These results are encouraging, but I should emphasize that the results are still preliminary and not yet final. Longer follow-up is definitely warranted to determine the impact of this therapeutic approach on long-term survival and ultimate salvage laryngectomy, as well as on quality of life. These results cannot yet be directly applied as suggesting a treatment modality for other head and neck cancer sites.

Future developments

Based on the experience of the VA Laryngeal Cancer Study Group, we now need to design some further studies, with 3 aims. First, local control must be improved. We might be able to do this by using hyperfractionation XRT after chemotherapy or concurrent chemotherapy and XRT, either upfront or after induction chemotherapy. One trial presented at the 1989 ASCO meeting studied patients who did not respond to induction chemotherapy, were given concurrent cisplatin and radiation therapy, and then showed a high complete response rate. This was an interesting result and this strategy should be considered for further study, possibly alternating chemotherapy and radiation therapy to improve local control.

Our second aim should be to decrease distant metastases. I am convinced from our study and those from the Head and Neck Contract Group and Dr Frei's group at the Dana-Farber Institute that distant metastases can be decreased with more traditional adjuvant chemotherapy, especially in responders.

Effective chemoprevention strategies to decrease secondary cancers must be developed, especially if we are considering long-term survivors.

It is important to determine whether similar approaches are feasible for tumors arising from other head and neck sites where humiliating and debilitating surgery is often performed. Several studies are already addressing this issue: Dimery and colleagues at the M.D. Anderson Cancer Center in Houston, in collaboration with surgeons and diagnostic radiologists, have been investigating combined intraarterial chemotherapy with systemic chemotherapy in patients with advanced head and neck or sinus cancer.

Finally, it is well understood that quality of life is a very important issue, especially in the treatment of head and neck cancer patients. However, it is important not to trade survival for quality of life. The ideal goal is to improve both survival and quality of life at the same time.

References

1. Cancer Statistics—1988. New York: American Cancer Society; 1988.
2. Hong WK, Bromer R. Medical intelligence. Current concepts: Chemotherapy in head and neck cancer. N Engl J Med 1983;308:75–9.
3. Clark JR, Fallon BG, Frei E III. Induction chemotherapy as initial treatment for advanced head and neck cancer: A model for multidisciplinary treatment of solid tumors. In: DeVita V, Hellman S, Rosenberg S, eds. Oncology 1987. Philadelphia: Lippincott; 1987:175–9.

4. Wittes R, Heller K, Randolph V, et al. Cis-dichlorodiammineplatinum (II)-based chemotherapy as intitial treatment of advanced head and neck cancer. Cancer Treat Rep 1979;63:1533–8.

5. Randolph VL, Vallejo AM, Spiro RH, et al. Combination therapy of advanced head and neck cancer: Induction of remissions with diamminedichloroplatinum (II), bleomycin and radiation therapy. Cancer 1978;41:460–7.

6. Hong WK, Bhtuani R, Shapsay SM, et al. Induction chemotherapy of advanced previously untreated squamous cell head and neck cancer with cisplatin and bleomycin. In: Preytayko A, Crooke S, Carter S, eds. Cisplatin: Current status and new developments. San Diego: Academic; 1980:431–44.

7. Jacobs C, Goffinet DR, Goffinet L, et al. Chemotherapy as a substitute for surgery in the treatment of advanced resectable head and neck cancer. Cancer 1987;60:1178–83.

8. Glick JH, Marcial V, Richter M, et al. The adjuvant treatment of inoperable stage III and IV epidermoid carcinoma of the head and neck with platinum and bleomycin infusions prior to definitive radiotherapy: An RTOG pilot study. Cancer 1980;46:1919–24.

9. Hill BT, Price LA. Induction combination chemotherapy without cisplatin followed by radiotherapy without radical surgery as definitive treatment for advanced epidermoid carcinoma of the larynx. Second International Congress on Neo-Adjuvant Chemotherapy, Paris, February 19–21, 1988. Abstract

10. Ensley JF, Jacobs JR, Weaver A, et al. The correlation between response to cis-platinum combination chemotherapy and subsequent radiotherapy in previously untreated patients with advanced squamous cell cancers of the head and neck. Cancer 1984;54:811–4.

11. Hong WK, O'Donoghue GM, Sheetz S, et al. Sequential response patterns to chemotherapy and radiotherapy in head and neck cancer: Potential impact of treatment in advanced laryngeal cancer. In: Wagener DJT, Blijham GH, Smeets JBE, et al, eds. Primary chemotherapy in cancer medicine. New York: Alan R. Liss; 1985:191–7.

12. Head and Neck Contracts Program. Adjuvant chemotherapy for advanced head and neck squamous carcinoma: Final report of the Head and Neck Contracts Program. Cancer 1987;60:301–11.

13. Schuller DE, Wilson H, Hodgson S, et al. Preoperative reductive chemotherapy for stage III or IV operable epidermoid carcinoma of the oral cavity, oropharynx, hypopharynx, or larynx, phase III. A Southwest Oncology Group Study. Proceedings of the International Conference on Head and Neck Cancer: Chemotherapy II, Baltimore, July 22–27, 1984. Abstract

14. Toohill RJ, Anderson T, Byhardt RW, et al. Cisplatin and fluorouracil as neoadjuvant therapy in head and neck cancer. Arch Otolaryngol Head Neck Surg 1987;113:758–61.

15. Stell PM, Dalby JE, Strickland P, et al. Sequential chemotherapy and radiotherapy in advanced head and neck cancer. Clin Radiol 1983;34:463–7.

16. Kun LE, Toohill RJ, Holoye PY, et al. A randomized study of chemotherapy for cancer of the upper aerodigestive tract. Int Radiat Oncol Biol Phys 1986;12:173–8.

17. Martin M, Mazeron JJ, Glaubiger D, et al. Neoadjuvant polychemotherapy of head and neck cancer: Preliminary results of a randomized study. Proc Am Soc Clin Oncol 1986;5:151. Abstract

18. Wolf GT, Makuch RW, Baker SR. Predictive factors for tumor response to preoperative chemotherapy in a patient with head and neck squamous carcinoma: The Head and Neck Contract Group. Cancer 1984;54:2869–77.

19. Pennacchio JL, Hong WK, Shapsay S, et al. Combination of cisplatinum and bleomycin prior to surgery and/or radiotherapy compared with radiotherapy alone for the treatment of advanced squamous cell carcinoma of the head and neck. Cancer 1982;50:2795–80.

20. Al-Sarraf M, Reading B, Kishj JA, et al. Adjuvant chemotherapy for patients with locally advanced head and neck cancer: RTOG and Wayne State University experience. In: Salmon SE, ed. Adjuvant therapy of cancer V. Philadelphia: Grune & Stratton; 1987: 89–100.

21. McNeil BJ, Werchelbaum R, Panker SG. Speed and survival: Tradeoffs between quality and quantity of life in laryngeal cancer. N Engl J Med 1981;305:982–7.

22. Karp D, Carter R, Vaughan C, et al. Voice preservation using induction chemotherapy plus radiation therapy as an alternative to laryngectomy in advanced head and neck cancer: Long-term follow-up. Proc Am Soc Clin Oncol 1988;7:152. Abstract

23. Haines I, Bosl GJ, Pfister D, et al. Very high-dose cisplatin with bleomycin infusion as initial treatment of advanced head and neck cancer. J Clin Oncol 1987;5:1594–1600.

24. Hong WK, Wolf GT, Fisher S, et al. Laryngeal preservation with induction chemotherapy and radiotherapy in the treatment of advanced laryngeal cancer: Interim survival data of VACSP #268. Proc Am Soc Clin Oncol 1989;8:167. Abstract 650

Discussion

Chairperson: **Yukio Inuyama**

Dr Naoyuki Kohno (Metropolitan Otsuka Hospital, Tokyo): First I would like to ask you about induction chemotherapy. I think it is most important to obtain survival benefit, that is, to increase the CR rate. To do this, which is the most effective method, for example, increasing dose intensity?

Dr Hong: I think intensity of both chemotherapy and XRT are important in improving the CR rate. Unfortunately, there is a limit to the XRT dose, up to 7000 rad, due to toxicity, such as spinal cord damage or neck fibrosis, unless we modify the XRT dose and schedule. Therefore, dose intensity of chemotherapy is important in achieving a higher response and XRT can be very effective in controlling small tumors.

Dr Kohno: Maintenance chemotherapy is very important to reduce distant metastases. Do you have any comment about the schedule and period of maintenance chemotherapy?

Dr Hong: Again, there have been 3 studies addressing that issue. The first study was from the Head and Neck Contract Group. Their study was a 3-arm study of surgery and radiation therapy: the 2nd arm was induction chemotherapy followed by surgery/radiation, and the 3rd arm was induction chemotherapy, then surgery, radiation, and maintenance therapy. The induction regimen they used was cisplatin and bleomycin and, as maintenance chemotherapy, cisplatin alone as a single agent for 6 cycles after surgery and radiation treatment. There was no survival benefit in any of those 3 arms; however, the patients who received maintenance chemotherapy showed a reduction in distant metastases, so there is some benefit. Distant metastases were definitely decreased in patients who received maintenance chemotherapy; it was a positive study in that respect. The 2nd study was conducted by Dr Ervin at the Dana-Farber Cancer Institute. Patients who showed a response with induction chemotherapy then received the standard treatment, which is surgery and/or radiation therapy; the responders were then randomized to receive either additional chemotherapy or no further chemotherapy. The patients who received additional chemotherapy showed a reduction in distant metastases, compared to the patients who did not receive further maintenance chemotherapy. That was a positive study. The 3rd study that I mentioned is the VA Laryngeal Study Group. Although we did not give additional adjuvant chemotherapy after definitive treatment, the patients who received induction therapy had a decrease in distant metastases.

Dr Kohno: How long was the period?

Dr Hong: The Head and Neck Contract Group study in fact shows some problems with patient compliance in completing maintenance chemotherapy. Again, these are the types of patients with whom we deal. I think that in the Head and Neck Contract Group study only 20% of patients completed 6 cycles of maintenance chemotherapy. So, I think if I design a study in the future, I would like to give 3 additional cycles, but not as much as 6 cycles, because of the very poor compliance.

Dr Kohno: So you think about 10 cycles is ideal?

Dr Hong: No. Give induction chemotherapy for 3 cycles, and then, after the surgery and/or radiation treatment, give 3 more cycles. So there will be a total of 6 cycles.

Dr Yukio Inuyama (Hokkaido University School of Medicine, Sapporo): So the optimal number may be around 10 cycles. In that case, what about toxicity, of cisplatin, for example?

Dr Hong: We do not know what the optimal cycle is for the induction treatment; we do not know the optimal treatment for postoperative, adjuvant treatment. My guess is 3 cycles upfront and 3 more cycles afterward, so a total of 6 cycles is adequate. I think a patient can manage the toxicity up to 6 cycles, especially as long-term platinum treatment induces neurotoxicity, but I think that cisplatin can be replaced by carboplatin. If we believe that carboplatin is as active as cisplatin, then you can avoid having some long-term platinum-induced neurotoxicity by giving carboplatin.

Dr Tadashi Nakashima (National Kyushu Cancer Center, Fukuoka): May I ask you about some basic problems in cancer chemotherapy? In cancer chemotherapy for head and neck cancer patients I sometimes recognize differences in the response rate between the head and neck metastases and the primary tumors. Have you had any similar experiences?

Dr Hong: In fact, in the Laryngeal Cancer Study that we conducted, we looked at the response patterns by site, such as primary tumors versus nodal tumors, and I believe that there is a more favorable response at the primary site than at the nodal site. Why, I do not know. I think it has to do with the tumor cell heterogeneity and also it is very difficult to assess in the nodal tumor whether or not the patient achieves a real complete response or a partial response, but I think we see a more favorable response at the primary site than at a nodular tumor.

Dr Nakashima: Do you have a strategy for that?

Dr Hong: That is only my opinion. We are interested in looking for more response at the primary site. Our goal is to preserve the organs. Any residual disease on the neck can be operated on. That is another reason why we look at response by primary versus nodal sites.

Dr Nakashima: The goal of chemotherapy is to prevent distant metastases and neck node metastases. Do you use the same protocol for glottic and supraglottic cancer?

Dr Hong: We use the same chemotherapy, which is platinum and 5FU, and we stratify by site, supraglottic versus glottic. As I mentioned in my presentation, both groups are extremely well balanced.

Dr Hitoshi Saito (Fukui Medical School, Fukui): I was encouraged by your result of the decrease of the distant metastases, but I was discouraged about the primary recurrence and you did not mention increasing the CR rate with immune therapy. How about the evaluation in the USA of combined immune therapy?

Dr Hong: I agree with your first comment; we are very encouraged to see the decrease of distant metastases on the one hand, and we are concerned about the failures at the local/regional sites in the chemotherapy/radiation group.

To answer your question about the contribution of adding biological therapy to chemotherapy to increase the complete response rate, we have done a study at the M.D. Anderson Cancer Center using cisplatin and 5FU with interleukin 2

(IL-2). The patients had refractory cancer, recurrent head and neck cancer, and were not previously untreated patients. Dr Dimery at the M.D. Anderson Cancer Center reported this result at the 1989 ASCO meeting. We treated over 35 patients and the overall response rate with chemotherapy with IL-2 was 35%, which is no better than with chemotherapy alone. The complete response rate we obtained from that regimen was less than 10%. I must say that there is a lot of toxicity with IL-2, so we have closed that study now and we are developing a new study with cisplatin plus 5FU with interferon, because several studies have shown some synergystic activity of cisplatin with interferon and we will try to take advantage of that concept to improve the CR rate in head and neck cancer.

Dr Emil Frei III: In the postchemotherapy biopsies when the patients were in complete remission it was negative in 75%, which is good. I was a little surprised to see it negative in 50% of the PRs and 40% of the NRs. Would you comment on whether this is a technical problem with biopsies, or maybe we are really doing much better than we think in some of the PRs?

Dr Hong: I think that is a very good point. The tumor in the larynx, especially the glottic tumor, is not easily assessed by indirect examination. All the patients were examined under direct endoscopy by head and neck surgeons. Clinically there is some residual tumor and bulging out of the vocal cord and we did not call that a complete response. We biopsied those patients; clinically they appeared to have a partial response and from the biopsy it turned out that there was no tumor. Again, I would like to emphasize that there is some possible sampling error as well. A deep biopsy was not done; it was a very superficial biopsy. I think, especially in the evaluation of the tumor response in the larynx, not the oral cavity, indirect evaluation is not really an adequate way to evaluate the response.

Dr Frei: Did the partial responders with negative biopsy show better survival than partial responders with positive biopsy?

Dr Hong: This is because of the interim analysis. We have not really looked at subset analysis yet, but when we looked at the complete responders, the survivors versus the nonresponders, there was a definite survival benefit, but I think those are partial responders; when there was a negative tumor we did not look at the survival curve. One point I might add: the patients who received the 2-cycle induction chemotherapy showed no response. They underwent surgery and radiation treatment and we looked at those patients' survival. It is interesting that the survival of those patients is as good as in the patients who received upfront surgery and radiation treatment, but we need longer follow-up.

Breast cancer

Regulation of breast cancer by secreted growth factors

Marc E. Lippman

Georgetown University Medical Center, Washington, D.C.

Introduction

Clinicians involved with the care of patients with breast cancer are aware that most current therapies often prove to be inadequate. This does not mean that there have been no worthwhile developments or benefits for patients through the use of treatments such as adjuvant chemotherapy, newer endocrine therapies, and, possibly, bone marrow transplantation. I would certainly not wish to suggest that continued application of these rational principles will not continue to benefit an increasing number of patients with breast cancer. However, a more fundamental understanding of some of the mechanisms underlying the growth of cancers in general, and breast cancers in particular, is needed. Certain principles need to be understood, which I believe underlie not only breast cancer, but which are probably also shared by many other epithelial cancers, for example, lung, colorectal, gastric, and prostate. It will be from such a base that new forms of therapy will be developed to combat these diseases.

We already have some knowledge of the ways in which human cancers are substantially affected or cured by therapies that have been biologically engineered toward mechanisms underlying the growth of cancer. The regulation of breast cancer by growth factors is one such potential biologically based therapy. For this to be developed we need to consider the following questions, using breast cancer as the model.

1) What is the evidence that growth factors, such as insulin, insulin-like growth factors, or any others, are actually growth factors for tumors in vivo, in patients with cancer? Is there any formal evidence for autocrine, paracrine, or endocrine loops involving these factors?

2) What evidence is there that growth factors are responsible for malignant behavior, compared simply with mitogenesis or growth?

3) The answers to 1) and 2) lead to the critical question, particularly for clinicians: Is there reasonable hope that sufficient specificity exists in the way

73

that growth factors promote cancer (tumorigenesis) so that they can then be used for clinical benefit?

4) If such specificity does exist, is it within ligands or growth factors, or is it in the coupling of intracellular mechanisms, by which the receptors signal cells to behave in a malignant fashion?

5) Finally, can drugs be found that have sufficient specificity to interfere with the growth pathways of cancer, but not normal cells?

To investigate these issues we used both isolated human breast cancer cells grown in a test tube or tissue culture, and human tumors reconstituted in experimental animals.

Evidence for growth factors in tumors

All breast cancer, at least initially, is known to be estrogen responsive. Women who never have functioning ovaries never develop breast cancer, therefore from a promotional point of view, estrogens are essential for tumorigenesis to develop. When seen clinically, however, breast cancers may or may not be hormone dependent, ie, estrogen responsive. Unfortunately, all breast cancer in the clinic eventually becomes hormone independent. The patients are either unresponsive to endocrine therapies when first seen, or they have become resistant after having antiestrogen treatment.

I believe that hormone-dependent breast cancer cells secrete potent growth factors that are responsible for tumor growth and progression. These may be either autocrine, autostimulatory, or paracrine, ie, able to stimulate surrounding cells. These will be able to interact with blood vessels, fibroblasts, and the stroma that surrounds the cells. The growth factors may be regulated strictly in a positive sense by estrogens and therefore negatively regulated by drugs such as antiestrogens. I would also add that hormone-independent breast cancer cells secrete identical growth factors but these factors are being produced in an unregulated or constitutive fashion. This is an important hypothesis since if it is true, a therapy directed against one of these growth factors could be potentially successful for the treatment of both hormone-dependent and -independent breast cancers (Table 1).

As a first principle, I suggest that estrogens directly interact with the genome of human breast cancer cells, thereby altering gene expression. This eventually leads to tumor growth, invasion, and metastases. A huge number of enzymes involved in DNA synthesis can be shown to be regulated by estrogens and estrogens clearly interact directly with the genome to induce, at the level of gene transcription, many enzymes involved in growth. I believe the growth factors are necessary, and a sufficient condition for the induction of tumors and the following experiments support this.

Human breast cancers will grow as tumors in the flanks of athymic nude mice, and if these are hormone-dependent tumors, they will only grow if the animals

Table 1   Basic hypotheses for the roles of growth factors in breast cancer.

I.	Estrogens directly interact with the genome of human breast cancer to alter gene expression
II.	Hormone-dependent human breast cancer cells secrete potent autocrine and paracrine growth factors which are regulated by estrogens and antiestrogens and are responsible for tumor growth and progression
III.	Hormone-independent human breast cancers secrete identical autocrine and paracrine growth factors in a constitutive fashion
IV.	Antiestrogens inhibit breast cancer growth by inhibition of numerous cellular activities, including secretion of growth factors *and* by direct stimulation of RNA and protein products with inhibitory function

receive estrogen supplementation. Therefore, if estrogens produce tumors by inducing growth factor production, we ought to see tumor formation in these mice when we give growth factors produced by breast cancer cells rather than estrogens. When this experiment is carried out we find this to be true. That is, growth factors produced by breast cancer cells in culture can completely replace estrogen to induce tumor formation. The actual tumors grown after treatment with growth factors are invasive adenocarcinomas which are histologically indistinguishable from the tumors produced by estrogen. We believe that this provides proof that growth factors produced by breast cancer cells are critical for human breast cancer development.

The role of growth factors

In discussing the following experiments relating to growth factor activities and their biological significance, I will be using our work done with transforming growth factor alpha (TGFα). This is a protein that spans the cell membrane and has a molecular weight of approximately 19 000. It can be specifically clipped by proteases to yield a 6000 molecular weight peptide that is secreted by the cell (Fig 1).

TGFα is called a transforming growth factor because it can induce normal cells to behave like cancer cells. The evidence we have for this transforming activity comes from fibroblast experiments. When normal fibroblasts are grown on soft agar they cannot form large colonies and are therefore described as anchorage dependent. Only cancerous cells can grow unattached to dish surfaces, ie, they are anchorage independent. When fibroblasts treated with TGFα from breast cancer cells are grown on soft agar they grow and form large colonies, a sign of malignant growth.

Other evidence for the importance of TGFα is found when determining its presence in patients with breast cancer. In clinical cases of breast cancer we find that two-thirds of the patients test positively for TGFα, whether or not they are

75

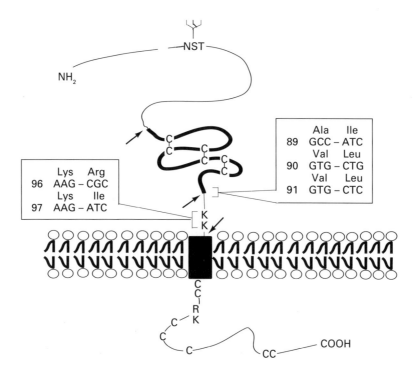

Fig 1   Structure of TGFα-derived peptide secreted by cancer cells.

hormone dependent. In fact, this number of about 70% is too low, because when the urine of patients is studied, 100% of them have elevated levels of TGFα-like activity.

Extra experimental evidence is also provided by RNA studies. We investigated whether messenger RNA, the precursor for TGFα, can be induced by estrogen treatment. It was found that physiological doses of estrogen can induce TGFα message, and that the protein is produced in breast cancer cells and is not an artifact of cells in culture.

Is TGFα responsible for mitogenesis or malignancy?

Since breast cancers produce TGFα, is this growth factor necessary for the development of the cancers? In order to answer this question, a mechanism of interfering with the activity of the growth factor had to be found. We did this in 2 ways. First, we used antibodies against the growth factor TGFα and determined whether they could interfere with the growth of human breast cancer cells. In culture experiments there was a dramatic reduction in the growth of breast cancer cell colonies when treated with such antibodies (Table 2).

Table 2   Effects of polyclonal anti-human TGFα antibody on MCF-7 human breast cancer cells.

	No. of colonies per dish
Control	677
+ Anti-h TGFα Ab	23
+ Preimmune rabbit IgG	640

A similar experiment was also done where the antibodies used were directed against the cell surface receptor to which the growth factors bind. In the culture experiments there was once again a significant inhibition of growth of tumors. The same results were obtained when the experiments were carried out in the nude mouse, ie, when they were treated with antibodies there was a prevention of tumor formation. Such experiments strongly suggest that autocrine or autostimulatory loops are essential for the growth of human breast cancers. This then led us to investigate whether the growth factor TGFα played an important role in transforming normal breast to malignant breast cells.

We introduced into hormone-dependent breast cancer cells a synthetic gene that would express TGFα. We then studied what happened to these cells, which had previously required estrogen stimulation to become malignant. Would they now, through the production of TGFα, become malignant without the stimulation of estrogen? We found that in cells with an induced high level of TGFα, due to incorporation of this synthetic gene, they still would not form tumors in the absence of estrogens, but in the presence of estradiol they would (Fig 2). This

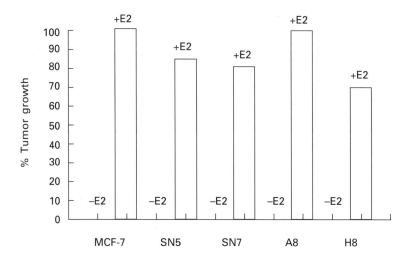

Fig 2   Growth of tumors in nude mice.

showed that although the TGFα is required for tumor formation, the expression of this one factor is not, by itself, sufficient to convert these cells to become independent of estrogen. This experiment is therefore consistent with the suggestion that TGFα is only one of the growth factors produced by breast cancer cells.

TGFα has been detected in normal human milk and normal breast epithelium. It is also possible, using the technique of in situ hybridization, to detect the messenger RNA for TGFα. When this is done we see that the normal breast expresses huge amounts of TGFα and that most of it is localized to the epithelial cells lining the duct. We believe that TGFα contributes to the growth, not only of malignant breast cells, but also of normal epithelial cells. It is responsible for the mitogenesis of these cells, but not their transformation from normal to malignant.

It is also interesting to note that in the TGFα synthetic gene experiments the breast cancer cells actually began producing a TGFα-like substance which had a molecular weight of 30 000 rather than the expected 6000. We investigated this higher molecular weight form, purified it to homogeneity, and found it had a molecular mass of 30 000 with sugars added onto it. It is glycosylated when the sugars are removed, to a molecular mass of 22 000, which is entirely different from the expected result for TGFα. This molecule has now been successfully cloned and it appears that human breast cancer cells are producing a new member of the TGFα family, not produced by normal breast epithelium and cells. This also has different functions from normal TGFα and is currently under investigation.

It must be emphasized that TGFα can clearly stimulate the growth of breast cancer, is produced by essentially all women with breast cancer and in nude mice experiments the growth of breast cancers can be strongly inhibited, without toxicity, by interfering with TGFα through the use of antibodies.

Fibroblast growth factor

As TGFα does not transform epithelial cells to malignant cells, we investigated whether another factor could be identified that would contribute to malignant behavior. To do this a suitable assay system was needed. For this we used a human adrenal carcinoma cell line, SW-13. These cells grow well in an anchorage-dependent assay with a doubling time of $1\frac{1}{2}$ days. However, they do not grow spontaneously in soft agar (anchorage independent) and are not stimulated to grow in soft agar by epidermal growth factor (EGF), TGFs α or β, insulin, insulin-like growth factors, or platelet-derived growth factors. However, fibroblast growth factor (FGF) is capable of stimulating the carcinoma cells to grow in soft agar. FGF does not function as a growth factor for these cells, but has transforming activity. Evidence for this has come from the growth of the same type of cells in an anchorage-dependent assay. There is no effect at all on cell

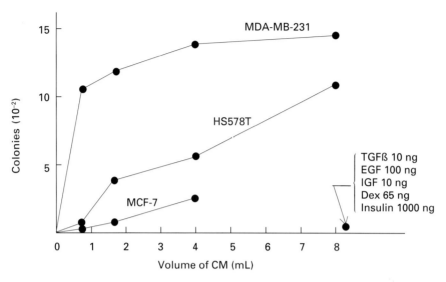

Fig 3   Production of an anchorage-dependent growth-stimulating activity for epithelial cells by human breast cancer cell lines.

growth rate if FGF is added. FGF appears to act by allowing these cells to acquire more malignant behavior, but it does not directly stimulate their growth.

We therefore attempted to determine whether there was a similar factor produced by breast cancer cells that would stimulate these cells to grow in soft agar. To do this we looked at about 50 human breast cancer cell lines (Fig 3). We also looked at about 9 human lung cancer cell lines, more than 25 colon cancer cell lines, and about 6 prostate cell lines. All of these cell lines produced a material that induced the SW-13 cells to form colonies in soft agar. This material was purified to homogeneity and found to be a 57 000–59 000 molecular weight dimer. As expected, this protein was capable of stimulating colony formation and, furthermore, the peak of activity on a radioreceptor assay competed with radioactive basic FGF (Fig 4). This suggested that this material was binding to FGF receptors and was therefore a new member of the FGF family.

FGF peptides are known to stimulate mesenchyme or mesodermal cells and to be angiogenic. It is also known that other cancers such as melanoma, hepatoma, and retinoblastoma can produce members of the FGF family. We attempted to show that production of this new growth factor transformed or contributed to the transformation of normal cells to malignant. To do this we introduced into the adrenal carcinoma cells a synthetic, FGF-like gene, K-FGF (Kaposi's sarcoma) which is identical to the *hst* (human stomach tumor) gene identified by Japanese investigators. The gene is stimulated by a cytomegalovirus (CMV) promoter. When the gene was introduced, the cells changed from being unable to grow in

79

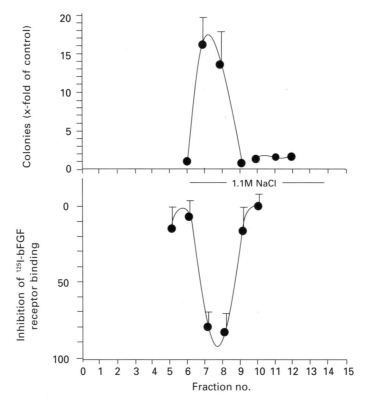

Fig 4 Inhibition of basic FGF-receptor binding and SW-13 cell soft agar stimulation by CM MDA-MB 231 after heparin affinity chromatography.

soft agar to forming colonies and from being nontumorigenic in nude mice to being rapidly fatal. In summary, the human adrenal carcinoma cells transfected with this FGF-like gene produced the expected mRNA, secreted the appropriate protein, grew in soft agar, and formed tumors in nude mice. Interestingly, when cultivated with normal nontransformed cells, they also stimulated these cells to grow in soft agar and in nude mice. This shows that normal cells can be transformed through a paracrine mechanism to behave in a malignant fashion.

Applications of FGF

If the growth factor FGF is responsible for malignant behavior, we could now look for a way to interfere with its activity and hence produce an important antitumor effect. We studied this in 2 ways: first, using a very toxic drug called suramin (a polysulfonated compound), which completely blocks tumor formation in soft agar; second, with an agent called pentosan, which can block the FGF-like activity at the receptor site. When we studied the growth of tumors in nude mice under controlled conditions, and when treated with pentosan, we found that tumor formation was completely inhibited. This agent was essentially nontoxic. We believe that such experiments provide evidence that, in vivo, tumor formation can be inhibited by growth factors and such therapies and by their receptor-binding action can achieve significant and nontoxic antitumor effects. We will therefore be shortly introducing pentosan into clinical trials.

Conclusions

A breast cancer cell, when stimulated by estrogens, produces a variety of growth factors. We have investigated the TGFα-like and FGF-like material. Many other growth factors can be produced, all of which can be shown to contribute to tumor formation. Furthermore, when tumors become hormone independent, these same growth factor activities are produced by breast cancer cells.

We have shown 3 different mechanisms which interfere with these growth factors: antibodies against the factors themselves; antibodies that block the receptor; and drugs that interfere with the association of the growth factor with the receptor. We believe that these experiments strongly suggest that growth factor activities are important in the pathogenesis of breast cancer. I would also like to speculate that many cancers which are morphologically readily distinguishable (lung, colon, rectal, prostate, and breast) have many similarities in terms of growth factor activities that they produce. Such secreted activities produced by cancer cells are essential, both for their growth and their malignant behavior, and therefore are attractive targets as potential antitumor agents for the future.

Further reading

Lippman ME, Dickson RB. Mechanisms of growth control in normal and malignant breast epithelium. Recent Progr Horm Res 1989;45:383–440.
Lippman ME, Dickson RB. Mitogenic regulation and malignant breast epithelium. Yale J Biol Med 1989;62:459–80.

Discussion

Chairperson: **Takeshi Tominaga**

Dr Yoshinobu Kubota (Yokohama City University School of Medicine, Yokohama): I understand your opinion that estrogen induces growth factor that is responsible for the malignant character of breast cancer. Is there any possibility that estrogen or other hormones induce growth factor receptors? Also, what relation is there between the *C-erb-1* gene expression of human breast cancer and the effect of estrogen?

Dr Lippman: It is important that you understand that, although I have shown evidence that estrogens can induce growth factors, I do not wish to imply that other important genetic events that can occur in these cells also play an important part in tumor formation. For example, it is possible to imagine that estrogens, as you suggested in your question, induce certain growth factor receptors and there has been some experimentation that has suggested that that can occur. For example, the EGF to which TGFα binds is overexpressed in human breast cancers that have more malignant behavior. We have also noticed that estrogens can turn off genes in cells that prevent more malignant behavior. For example, the MCF-7 cells, in the absence of estrogen, when they cannot grow, express high levels of *rb*, the retinoblastoma gene, and when they are treated with estrogens they increase their growth factor production, but they turn off fair expression of *rb*. We have recently found evidence that estrogen downregulates *rb*-B2. The mechanism of this regulation is under investigation.

Dr Masakazu Toi (Research Institute for Nuclear Medicine and Biology, Hiroshima University, Hiroshima): My first question is: I would like to know how FGF is expressed in human breast cancer tissues and what its messenger RNA level is? Is FGF related to estrogen receptor or hormone dependency?

Dr Lippman: There are several members of the FGF family that have already been identified and each of them has to be examined separately because RNA and antibody probes are different for each of them and we have just begun those experiments. Looking at a small series, perhaps 40–45 human breast cancers, we have thus far found FGF activity in all of them, but we have not yet performed immunocytochemistry or in situ hybridization that would allow us to be certain that this is being produced by the breast cells, compared with other surrounding cells. I hope to have more information about that soon, but I do not have any answers for that today.

Dr Toi: My second question is: I understand that FGF receptor blockers are very effective in SW-13 cells. Is this therapy applicable to other types of cancer, for example, gastrointestinal cancer?

Dr Lippman: We have only used these drugs which interfere with FGF-like activity on several of our breast cancer cell lines, and an assortment of tumors. We can block tumor formation in nude mice for some and we are very encouraged by that, but we have not yet looked at a large number of cell lines. Preliminarily, these data look good, but a lot more needs to be done.

Dr Michihiko Kuwano (Oita Medical College, Oita): My question is related to the expression of the *erb* gene in the breast cancer cell. Did you investigate whether estrogen can regulate EGF levels in breast cancer cells?

Dr Lippman: At least in the experiments that we have done, estrogens do not have a major effect on the EGF receptor. When the cells grow faster or are stimulated to grow by estrogens there is some increase in EGF receptor, perhaps 2–3 fold, not a very major effect. In an experiment that I did not have time to discuss, we have successfully introduced the EGF receptor into breast cancer cells that expressed 2000–3000 receptor sites per cell and have succeeded in stimulating those cells to express more than 1 000 000 EGF receptors per cell and we know that by binding experiments it is a completely functional receptor. When we overexpress the EGF receptor in those cells we cannot make those cells hormone independent alone, so that that is not enough. However, the work from several groups has shown that there is a consistent correlation with high expression of the EGF receptor and a poor prognosis in patients with breast cancer, and it also correlates with high S phase, as measured by flow cytometry.

Dr Kuwano: My second question is: you just suggested that EGF or basic FGF is secreted from breast cancer cells. As you know, these are very angiogenic factors, so could you tell, for example, in vivo, whether your experimental data will show that breast cancers with high secretion of EGF or basic FGF are highly angiogenic?

Dr Lippman: In the tumors that are induced in nude mice by the cells that overexpress FGF, those tumors are extremely angiogenic. They have evidence for large endothelial spaces filled with blood vessels. Although I have tried to suggest that FGF-like peptides can function as an autocrine growth factor on breast cancer cells in cell culture, I do not wish to exclude that an important role is as a paracrine activity to permit angiogenesis, as your question suggests.

Dr Yasuo Nomura (National Kyushu Cancer Center, Fukuoka): You have said that there are 2 different kinds of growth factors related to hormone dependency of breast cancer. So by measuring these growth factors or their receptors, is it possible to predict hormone dependency of breast cancer more accurately than with the conventional estrogen receptor assay?

Dr Lippman: That is an excellent question, but I do not have an answer to it. What is required to answer that question is to look now at a reasonable number of tumor biopsies by methods that will specifically identify these growth factors or their receptors in the tumor samples, and ask what the correlations may be with clinical behavior. It is not until we have been able to clone successfully both FGF activity and the new TGFα that we will even be able to do those experiments. We hope to be carrying out those experiments soon, but I have no answers for you today.

Dr Nomura: Would you comment on whether or not tamoxifen is able to synchronize the breast cancer cells for estrogen-primed chemotherapy? Is it available for the metastatic breast cancer patient as a routine treatment?

Dr Lippman: Some years ago we suggested that it might be possible to increase the efficacy of chemotherapy by attempting to synchronize tumors, and we actually performed a randomized study with more than 100 patients, comparing a synchronization strategy to the same chemotherapy without it. There were modest but significant advantages to the synchronization arm; there was an improved survival and improved duration of response. We have, furthermore, obtained data by flow cytometry, as have other investigators in Italy, that prove that you can increase the growth fraction of breast cancer cells by several different strategies involving estrogens, with or without prior antiestrogen treatment. I believe that this kind of approach will probably not achieve a major benefit, but I do think that there is clear evidence that you can alter growth rates of tumors with estrogens. It is our hope that the information that we are learning about growth factors produced by breast cancer may permit us to alter the growth of larger proportions of tumor populations and it may be that we do not have completely to stop breast cancer growth for a long time with therapies against growth factors, but that we might increase the therapeutic index of the drugs we already have by short-term use of a variety of growth factors. As a single example in work coming from elsewhere, others have been able to show that TGFβ can block the growth of the normal gastrointestinal tract and therefore very substantially prevent the GI toxicity of certain kinds of drugs and therefore they can use these kinds of tricks to increase the amount of cytotoxic chemotherapy being given. I think that this is another possible way in which growth factor therapies may have a role to play.

Dr Michael J. O'Connell: Dr Lippman, your presentation was a very clear presentation of the possible importance of growth factors in clinical oncology. I agree with that point of view and I can provide 2 clinical examples that would suggest that growth factor inhibition therapy may be of potential clinical value in other systems. The first is based upon our observations of the use of a drug somatostatin analogue for the treatment of metastatic neuroendocrine carcinomas, particularly carcinoid tumors. This agent inhibits the secretion of peptide hormones from neuroendocrine cells, but has also been shown to inhibit the production of a number of growth factors. In our patients with advanced carcinoid tumors, we have not only seen significant improvement in carcinoid syndrome due to inhibition of peptide hormone release, but very interestingly, a small proportion, perhaps 10–15% of patients, have had major reductions in tumor and of even more interest is an apparent significant prolongation in the time to progression, ie, a decrease in the growth rate of these neuroendocrine cells. We are currently testing that hypothesis in colorectal cancer by performing a randomized trial for patients with advanced metastatic disease who have no symptoms, where half the patients are receiving somatostatin analogue therapy and the other half are randomized controls receiving no specific treatment to see whether the inhibition of putative growth factors may result in a delay in tumor progression.

The second example comes from prostate cancer, where at the National Cancer Institute in Washington, Dr Meyers and others have used suramin for treating metastatic prostate cancer, with a very high rate of reported objective tumor response. We, and investigators at Memorial Sloan-Kettering and M.D. Anderson are about to embark upon a confirmatory trial to see whether we can confirm those results using suramin as a growth factor inhibitor type of therapy.

Dr Kazutake Kawakami (Tohoku University School of Medicine, Sendai): Do normal cells cultured with TGFα secrete growth factors themselves?

85

Dr Lippman: Generally speaking, normal epithelial cells in culture will produce some growth factor activities, particularly human mammary cells when cultured will produce TGFα. If one looks at normal fibroblasts from human beings, they do not produce growth factor activities, but when those cells are transformed by a variety of oncogenes, eg, *ras* or *myc*, and become malignant, they then acquire the ability to produce growth factors. In an experiment that I did not have time to tell you about today, but which we have previously published, we have taken hormone-dependent breast cancer cells which secrete low levels of growth factors and which are stimulated to produce more growth factors by estrogen. We have introduced into those breast cancer cells an oncogene that they do normally express, *ras*. Those cells, when treated with *ras,* become hormone independent and will form tumors in nude mice without estrogens. We have shown that they produce substantially increased levels of growth factor activity. Dr Gelmann in our laboratory has repeated those experiments in hormone-dependent human prostate cancer and has shown by the introduction of *ras* that these cells become androgen independent and produce increased amounts of growth factor activity. We believe that these experiments are consistent with the idea that increased growth factor production may allow more normal cells to behave in a more malignant fashion.

Gastrointestinal cancer

Clinical applications of chemotherapy in the management of colorectal cancer

Michael J. O'Connell

Mayo Clinic, Rochester, Minnesota

Introduction

This article will review 4 distinct aspects of the clinical application of chemotherapy for the treatment of patients with colorectal cancer. First, a summary of recent improvements in systemic chemotherapy for advanced metastatic disease, which will put the magnitude of this improvement into clinical perspective. Second, a discussion on the advantages and limitations of regional intraarterial chemotherapy for the commonly encountered problem of unresectable metastatic colorectal cancer confined to the liver. Third, an update on the current status of surgical adjuvant chemotherapy for patients with high-risk colon cancer. Finally, the use of chemotherapy combined with radiation therapy as surgical adjuvant treatment for patients with high-risk rectal cancer will be reviewed.

Systemic chemotherapy for advanced colorectal cancer

From a historical perspective, the fluorinated pyrimidines remain the compounds most active as single agents against this disease. We have had the most experience with fluorouracil (5FU), which will produce temporary partial responses in approximately 20% of patients. Although cytotoxic agents, such as mitomycin C and the nitrosoureas, have some degree of activity, none surpasses the meager effect of 5FU. Empirically derived regimens formulated by the simple combination of agents with some degree of antitumor activity have not been effective in improving treatment results. Any increases in tumor response rates are frequently overshadowed by an increase in toxicity and there has been no such regimen demonstrated to improve patient survival.

Biochemical modulation of 5FU with leucovorin

In the past several years a great scientific interest has developed in biochemical modulation as a mechanism to improve the therapeutic effect of 5FU. We define biochemical modulation as an alteration of tumor cell metabolism to produce selective enhancement of cytotoxicity against the tumor. The intent is to improve the therapeutic index, not simply to increase the potency of 5FU against both tumor and normal tissues. Leucovorin (LV), also known as citrovorum factor or folinic acid, can act as a biochemical modulating agent to enhance the cytotoxic effect of 5FU. 5FU is metabolized to 5-fluorodeoxyuridine monophosphate, which then binds with thymidylate synthetase (TS) in the presence of a reduced folate cofactor known as 5,10-methylene tetrahydrofolic acid. The administration of LV (Fig 1) increases the amount of reduced folates within the cell as the LV is actively transported into the cancer cell. With an increase in the amount of the reduced folate cofactor, the entire reaction is moved to the right, where a ternary complex is formed which effectively removes TS from the biochemical machinery of the cell and thereby inhibits DNA formation. This is the mechanism for production of the cytotoxic effect. There are abundant preclinical data from several laboratories to support this biochemical interaction, although the amount of LV required to produce optimal 5FU cytotoxicity varies, depending upon the model system under study.

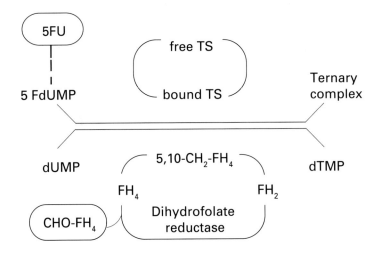

Fig 1   Biochemical interactions between 5FU and LV (CHO-FH$_4$).

In our experience with LV-modulated 5FU treatment for patients with advanced colorectal cancer [1] (the Mayo Clinic-North Central Cancer Treatment Study Group [NCCTG] study), patients with advanced metastatic disease were randomly assigned to receive treatment with one of several different chemotherapy regimens, 2 of which will be discussed here. We administered 5FU 500 mg/m^2 by iv push daily, for 5 consecutive days, with courses repeated every 5 weeks. This represents the maximum tolerated dose of 5FU that can safely be given to patients by this method, according to our experience. LV was added to 5FU at 2 distinct dose levels, based upon preclinical laboratory data and preliminary clinical experience: a high dose (200 mg/m^2) daily for 5 consecutive days, or a low dose (20 mg/m^2) for 5 consecutive days. The daily 5FU dose was 370 mg/m^2 when given with high-dose LV and we were able to increase the 5FU to 425 mg/m^2 daily when given with low-dose LV. The combined courses were repeated at 4 and 8 weeks, then every 5 weeks.

We found that objective tumor responses were seen significantly more frequently in patients receiving LV in combination with 5FU, in contrast to those patients receiving 5FU alone. We defined an objective tumor response as at least a 50% reduction in sum of the products of bidimensionally measurable indicator lesions or a greater than one-third reduction in the linear measurement of palpable hepatomegaly. These responses had to be observed at least 8 weeks following the initiation of treatment. Ten percent of 39 patients receiving 5FU alone experienced an objective tumor response compared with 26% of 35 patients receiving 5FU plus high-dose LV and 43% of 37 patients treated with 5FU and low-dose LV. The objective response rates associated with each of the LV regimens were statistically superior to 5FU alone ($p < 0.04$, 5FU + high-dose LV; $p < 0.001$, 5FU + low-dose LV) and there was no statistical difference between the 2 LV regimens.

The quality of life of patients undergoing palliative chemotherapy is an important clinical endpoint. We therefore examined the frequency of symptomatic improvement in tumor-related symptoms, increase in weight, and improvement in performance status for patients undergoing therapy. In each case there was a statistically significant improvement in the proportion of patients experiencing benefit with 5FU plus low-dose LV compared to 5FU alone. Symptomatic improvement was 34% of 38 patients given 5FU alone, 40% of 42 patients given 5FU + high-dose LV, and 69% of 36 patients given low-dose LV ($p < 0.05$ vs controls). The patients treated with 5FU and high-dose LV experienced improvement in 2 of the 3 parameters compared to the controls.

There were approximately 70 patients in each treatment group, of whom about 90% had died at the time of analysis for survival experience (Fig 2). There was a significant improvement in survival among patients treated with either of the LV-containing regimens as compared to 5FU alone. Median survival was increased from approximately 7 months with 5FU alone, to approximately 12 months with the addition of LV. Although survival was prolonged, there was no evidence of a curative effect, since the survival curves came together at 2 years.

The improvement in therapeutic effect just reviewed was not observed at the expense of an increase in severe toxicity. About two-thirds (67%) of 70 patients treated with single-agent 5FU experienced one or more severe chemotherapy side

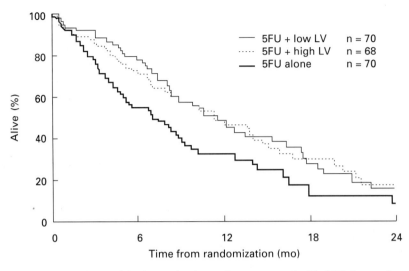

Fig 2 Survival of patients with advanced colorectal cancer treated with 5FU alone or in combination with high-dose or low-dose LV (NCCTG).

effects. Fifty-seven percent of 68 and 56% of 70 patients, respectively receiving 5FU + high-dose or low-dose LV experienced this degree of chemotherapy toxicity. Thus, since the therapeutic effect was improved against the cancer without an increase in toxicity against normal tissue, an improvement in therapeutic index has been demonstrated when LV is added to 5FU. However, the pattern of toxicity of 5FU is markedly altered when LV is added. Leucopenia is the dose-limiting toxicity of loading course bolus 5FU, with 48% of 70 patients in this study experiencing a white blood count nadir of <2000. Only approximately 20% of patients receiving 5FU + LV (19% and 21% of patients given additional high-dose LV or low-dose LV, respectively) experienced this degree of hematologic toxicity. On the other hand, stomatitis was the dose-limiting toxicity with the 5FU + LV regimens and was seen in about one-third of patients (30% of 68 patients [p<0.05] given high-dose LV and 26% of 70 patients given low-dose LV [p<0.05]), significantly more frequent than seen with 5FU alone. Severe diarrhea was not seen more frequently with these loading course 5FU + LV regimens.

Other investigators have examined different schedules of chemotherapy administration, including weekly treatment, different doses of 5FU ranging from 370 to 600 mg/m^2, and different doses and duration of LV infusions ranging to as high as 500 mg/m^2 by continuous 24-h infusion. The toxicity profiles showed that ulcerative stomatitis is the dose-limiting toxicity of 5FU + LV regimens when 5FU is given by the loading course technique. On the other hand, severe diarrhea is the dose-limiting toxicity with weekly administration. This diarrhea can produce a profuse cholera-like syndrome which, if not recognized and vig-orously treated, can lead to dehydration and death. Significantly less myelosup-pression is observed with either method of 5FU + LV administration compared to single agent 5FU given at its maximum tolerated dose by iv push.

Six of 7 randomized clinical trials have indicated a significant improvement in tumor response rate with 5FU + LV chemotherapy compared to single agent 5FU. Short-term survival has been prolonged in 2 of the 7 trials, including our own. Based on our results, and those of others reported in literature, we conclude that 5FU combined with LV represents a true therapeutic advance in the treatment of advanced colorectal cancer. Tumor response rates have been doubled to the 30–40% range and median survival has been improved by approximately 5 months in our experience. It should be recognized, first, that the magnitude of improvement and therapeutic effect is relatively small and therefore continuing emphasis on clinical research to provide even more effective therapy is certainly indicated. Second, the efficacy results obtained in our study with 5FU + high-dose LV and 5FU + low-dose LV were indistinguishable, ie, when combined with intensive course 5FU, there appears to be no advantage to the use of daily LV doses above 20 mg/m². We are currently comparing a high-dose weekly 5FU + LV regimen versus the low-dose LV intensive-course regimen discussed above, to further define the optimal dosage administration schedule for clinical practice. We are also in the process of combining 5FU + LV chemotherapy with radiation treatment, and studying this combination in the surgical adjuvant setting, where we hope that a significant impact on long-term survival may be possible in the minimal tumor burden setting afforded following resection of a primary colon cancer.

Regional intraarterial therapy for unresectable colorectal liver metastases

The liver is an organ commonly involved in hematogenous metastases from colorectal cancer, and liver failure is a frequent cause of death. There is a rationale for the intraarterial route of chemotherapy administration for some cytotoxic agents to treat this problem. A higher regional drug concentration can be achieved for drugs with rapid total body clearance and a high extraction ratio by the liver. This increase in drug delivery should provide an enhanced cytotoxic effect based upon dose-response relationships. A decrease in systemic toxicity would be anticipated if there is a high rate of extraction of the drug on the first pass through the hepatic arterial circulation, since very little drug would reach the systemic circulation.

An implantable infusion pump provides the technology to administer reliably prolonged continuous intraarterial infusions with low rates of sepsis or bleeding, 2 complications frequently observed with the transcutaneous use of temporary angiographically placed catheters. The catheter tip is placed in the hepatic arte-rial circulation at the time of laparotomy. The pump is implanted beneath the skin of the abdominal wall, creating a completely closed system within the body. Using this technique to administer 5-fluorodeoxyuridine (5FUdR) for colorectal liver metastases, a wide range of objective tumor responses has been reported from various investigators ranging from as high as 80% in the 1983 Alabama study to as low as 20% in the 1985 Chicago study (Fig 3). Differences in response criteria and patient selection factors likely account for this wide variation in these uncontrolled trials.

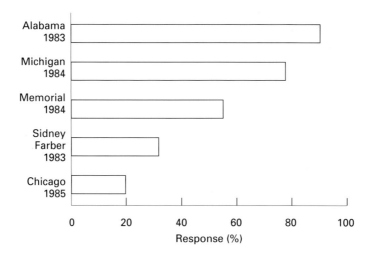

Fig 3 Summary of objective response rates in uncontrolled trials of intraarterial FUdR for treatment of colorectal liver metastases.

We have recently completed a controlled trial of intrahepatic 5FUdR compared to a standard regimen of intravenous 5FU [2]. Patients with colorectal cancer clinically confined to the liver were stratified according to their performance status, extent of hepatic metastases, and the presence or absence of a measurable indicator lesion, and were then randomized to receive one of the treatment regimens. FUdR 0.3 mg/kg was administered by continuous intraarterial infusion for 14 days each month. 5FU 500 mg/m^2 was given as an intravenous bolus for 5 consecutive days at 5-weekly intervals. We observed a significantly (p<0.01) higher tumor response rate with intrahepatic therapy than with systemic therapy. Fifty-four percent of 26 patients receiving intrahepatic treatment versus 21% of 29 patients receiving systemic treatment had at least a 50% reduction in the size of the hepatic metastases. Furthermore, the time to progression of malignant disease within the liver was significantly better for patients with intrahepatic therapy (Fig 4). However, intrahepatic therapy did not improve the overall time to progression of malignant disease which includes sites other than the liver (Fig 5). There was also no evidence of prolongation of survival for patients receiving intrahepatic therapy.

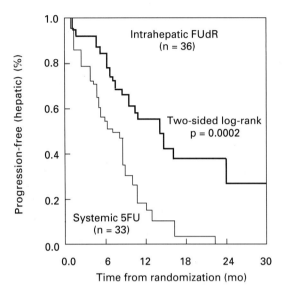

Fig 4   Time to progression of malignant disease within the liver in patients treated with intrahepatic FUdR or systemic 5FU (Mayo Clinic-NCCTG).

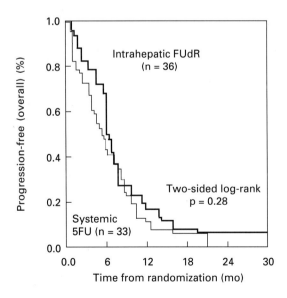

Fig 5   Overall time to progression of malignant disease in patients treated with intrahepatic FUdR or systemic 5FU (Mayo Clinic-NCCTG).

Three other randomized trials, comparing intrahepatic 5FUdR with systemic infusions of this agent, have been reported in the USA (Table) [3–6]. In each case there was a significantly higher response rate of tumor within the liver associated with the use of intrahepatic therapy. None of the studies, however, demonstrated improved survival, due to failure to control progression of malignant disease outside the liver. In addition, jaundice due to chemical hepatitis (24%), gastritis or ulceration due to inadvertent perfusion of the upper gastrointestinal tract (21%), and biliary strictures due to a direct toxic effect of 5FUdR on the bile ducts (9%) have been reported. These can be very severe or fatal if not recognized and managed appropriately.

Table   Summary of randomized trials of intrahepatic versus systemic chemotherapy for the treatment of colorectal liver metastases.

Study	Ref no.	Patients	Response (%)		Survival
Memorial	[3]	99	50 / 20	p=0.001	No
NCOG	[4]	110	37 / 10	p=0.002	No
NCI	[5]	64	62 / 17	p=0.003	No
Mayo/NCCTG	[6]	69	54 / 21	p=0.01	No

From these studies we conclude that intrahepatic chemotherapy with 5FUdR can significantly improve both the frequency and duration of tumor response in the liver, compared to systemic therapy with 5FU or 5FUdR. However, such treatment does not prevent tumor progression in extrahepatic sites and does not improve time to overall progression or patient survival. Our current research interest in this area is to combine intrahepatic therapy with systemic chemotherapy with the dual purpose of controlling tumor within the liver and preventing or delaying progression of malignant disease in extrahepatic sites. Intrahepatic therapy is not given in our medical practice outside a research protocol.

Adjuvant chemotherapy for resectable primary colon cancer

Patients at high risk for recurrence following surgery for colon cancer are identified using the modified Astler Coller staging system. Patients at high risk are those whose tumor has spread to regional lymph nodes and those with transmural penetration through the bowel wall, particularly when associated with an intestinal obstruction or perforation, or invasion of adjacent organs. These categories of patients are considered appropriate candidates for studies of adjuvant chemotherapy given following complete gross resection of the primary tumor. The aim is to eradicate occult metastatic disease and thereby increase the long-term survival or cure rates.

When evaluating clinical trials of surgical adjuvant chemotherapy for colorectal cancer, several clinical variables need to be borne in mind. First, colon cancer must be distinguished from rectal cancer, since rectal cancers much more frequently recur locally within the pelvis and therefore there is a much greater rationale for the use of combined chemotherapy and radiation therapy for this category of patients. Second, it should be noted whether chemotherapy is given as a single modality, which is the usual case for colon cancer, or combined with radiation therapy, which is being given with increased frequency for rectal cancer. Finally, the route of chemotherapy administration must be considered; for example, regional perfusion of the portal vein versus systemic intravenous therapy.

Several statistical variables are also of critical importance in evaluating the effect of adjuvant therapy. The use of prospectively randomized controls has been established as a prerequisite for adequate evaluation of an experimental therapy. A large enough sample size and long enough follow-up of patients must be available. Data quality must be high, ideally with fewer than 5% of patients excluded from effective analysis due to ineligibility or other protocol violations. Finally, definitive results must be based upon analysis of the overall randomized population, rather than on an arbitrarily selected subset of patients chosen after completion of the study.

One large trial conducted by the National Surgical Adjuvant Breast and Bowel Project (NSABP) in the USA suggested a small, but statistically significant benefit for 5FU + methyl lomustine + vincristine as adjuvant therapy for colon cancer. However, collected data from other studies (by the Gastrointestinal Tumor Study Group [GITSG], Veterans Administration Surgical Adjuvant Group, South West Oncology Group, Eastern Cooperative Oncology Group, and Cross Cancer Center), involving more than 2000 patients, indicated no significant survival advantage using this regimen and therefore we do not recommend this combination chemotherapy in this setting.

A different treatment approach using regional administration of chemotherapy into the portal vein during the perioperative period was developed in the UK by Taylor and colleagues. They recognized the frequent problem of liver metastases in patients with colon carcinoma and suggested that administration of chemotherapy by the same route into the portal circulation, the same route by which the tumor cells traverse from the colon to the liver, might be effective in eradicating microscopic foci of tumor before implantation and growth could occur. Perioperative treatment was favored to combat tumor implantation, facilitated by the stress of anesthesia and bowel manipulation.

The clinical trial performed by Taylor et al based on the above rationale was reported in 1985 [7]. Patients undergoing complete resection of a colorectal cancer were randomized to postoperative observation or a 7-day course of treatment with portal vein 5FU. A significant reduction in liver metastases was observed in patients receiving portal vein perfusion (4.2%) compared to those receiving surgery alone (17.3%). A statistically significant improvement in survival was also seen among patients receiving portal vein 5FU. However, a clinical trial by Mayo Clinic researchers and the North Central Cancer Treatment Group, reported at the 1989 meeting of the Society of Surgical Oncology [8], failed to reproduce these results. Two hundred and nineteen evaluable patients were randomized and treated according to the protocol of Taylor et al, but no decrease in the frequency of hepatic metastases with the use of portal vein 5FU could be demonstrated (a 12% incidence in liver metastases in patients who received portal vein infusion compared to 13% of patients who received surgery alone). Similarly, there was no indication of a positive effect on patient survival. Therefore, based on our experience, we do not recommend this method of adjuvant therapy. We will await with interest the results from several other prospectively randomized trials using this methodology which are currently under way in the USA, Europe, Australia, and Asia.

Recently there has been much interest in levamisole as an adjuvant treatment for colon cancer [9]. Levamisole is currently administered as an anthelminthic agent, but it also has immunostimulative properties. Based upon early work performed by Verhagen in Europe, the Mayo Clinic and the NCCTG initiated a 3-arm randomized trial to evaluate the effect of levamisole given alone or in combination with 5FU compared to surgery alone for high-risk colon cancer. Approximately 400 patients were entered into this trial. The results indicate a significant improvement in recurrence-free survival, particularly associated with the use of levamisole + 5FU compared to the controls (Fig 6). When data from only the patients who relapsed are examined, it can been seen that treatment with levamisole + 5FU provides a significant delay in relapse compared to surgery alone or surgery followed by levamisole without 5FU. However, no statistically significant improvement in overall survival can be demonstrated and therefore although the results are promising, they are not conclusive. If survival in the subset of patients with regional lymph node metastases (Dukes C classification) is examined, there is a statistically significant survival advantage associated with adjuvant therapy. When these data are subjected to a multivariate (Cox) model, this difference for the controls versus the levamisole + 5FU group is highly significant (Fig 7). However, we do not consider such a subset analysis to be definitive, rather we view such analysis as exploratory in the sense of generating a hypothesis to be tested in a confirmatory trial. Thus a 2nd national intergroup trial within the USA has been conducted in over 1400 patients [10]. This study separately randomized patients with regional lymph node metastases (Dukes C classification) from those with transmural penetration alone and provided a much larger sample size to detect any treatment effect more adequately.

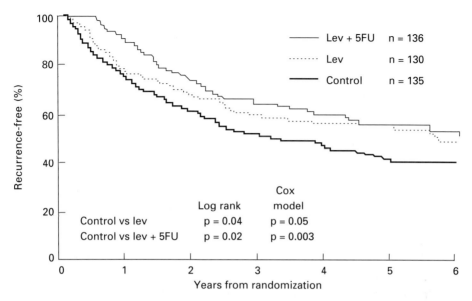

Fig 6 Recurrence-free survival for patients with resectable colorectal cancer, according to method of postoperative adjuvant therapy (NCCTG). Lev, levamisole.

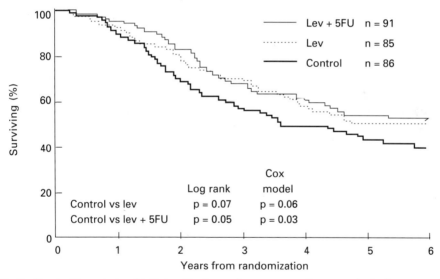

Fig 7 Survival in patients with Dukes C colorectal cancer, according to method of postoperative adjuvant therapy (NCCTG). Lev, levamisole.

Follow-up is presently not long enough to allow final analysis of the intergroup confirmatory trial and therefore we cannot recommend levamisole + 5FU as adjuvant therapy for colon cancer at the time of writing. However, if the confirmatory trial validates the promising results from our earlier study, this method of treatment would establish a new standard of care as surgical adjuvant therapy for patients with high-risk colon cancer.*

According to our current research protocol for surgical adjuvant therapy of colon cancer, patients are randomly assigned to surgery or chemotherapy with 5FU + LV following 2 different treatment schedules. Approximately 350 patients are currently registered to this protocol, but no results are available yet.[†]

Adjuvant therapy for rectal cancer

Since the rectum is located largely below the peritoneal reflection, there is no serosal barrier to prevent the direct extension of tumor cells into the perirectal tissues. These local tumor failures cause a great deal of distress to patients due to pain, pelvic abscesses, and urinary dysfunction. It has been shown that actual patient months of symptoms due to local tumor recurrence within the pelvis account for a much longer period of symptomatology compared to the effect of distant metastases. Rectal cancer can, of course, metastasize to distant sites, including the liver and lung, and therefore optimal adjuvant therapy should prevent both local tumor recurrence and distant metastasis. Studies have demonstrated that the addition of 5FU to radiation therapy can significantly improve local tumor control for patients with locally unresectable rectal carcinoma. A randomized trial reported by Moertel in 1970 in which patients with unresectable or recurrent rectal cancer receiving radiation therapy were randomized to receive also either concomitant administration of saline placebo or injections of 5FU showed a significant improvement in time to progression and survival among patients receiving both 5FU and radiation therapy.

Based on these principles, the GITSG conducted a randomized trial of postoperative adjuvant therapy for high-risk rectal cancer [11,12]. Patients received either observation, radiation therapy alone, chemotherapy alone, or the combination of radiation therapy + 5FU followed by systemic chemotherapy with methyl lomustine + 5FU. A significant advantage in disease-free survival was noted for patients treated with combined radiation and chemotherapy compared to surgery alone. Neither chemotherapy nor radiation therapy as a single modality had a significant treatment effect (Fig 8).

We subsequently conducted a 2nd rectal surgical adjuvant protocol comparing sequential chemotherapy plus radiation versus high-dose radiation therapy alone

---

*The national USA Intergroup Trial of levamisole with or without 5FU as adjuvant therapy for colon cancer has subsequently confirmed a highly significant decrease in tumor recurrence and death rates in patients with Dukes C tumors [6].

[†]This protocol has been terminated due to the positive results with 5FU + levamisole. We are currently using 5FU + levamisole as the control and studying a 3-day levamisole + leucovorin 5FU regimen and also testing different durations of adjuvant chemotherapy (6 versus 12 months).

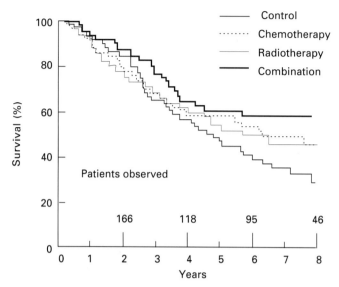

Fig 8 Survival for patients with rectal cancer, according to method of postoperative adjuvant therapy (GITSG).

[13]. The total treatment duration was decreased to 6 months in our trial compared with 18 months in the GITSG study. Once again, combined modality treatment provided a significant improvement in disease-free survival compared to the controls, with over 100 patients in each group. Likewise the addition of chemotherapy produced a significant survival advantage compared to the use of radiation alone and these differences have presently reached statistical significance.

Our current protocol is comparing 4 different methods of sequential combined modality therapy for patients with high-risk rectal cancer. We are addressing 2 issues. First, is it possible to decrease the toxicity of adjuvant therapy by deleting methyl lomustine, a chemotherapeutic agent associated with significant gastrointestinal and hematologic side effects and the potential for delayed acute leukemia? Second, we are also attempting to improve the effectiveness of combined modality therapy by studying a new method of 5FU administration as a radiation sensitizer during treatment with radiation therapy. Patients receive 5FU either by protracted venous infusion using a central venous catheter, or treatment with simple iv bolus therapy, as has been our practice in the past. Over 200 patients have entered this trial which is in progress as a national intergroup trial within the USA.

Future research

We believe that the priorities for future research in the surgical adjuvant therapy of colorectal cancer are as follows. First, more effective systemic therapies must be developed. Regimens based on the principles of biochemical modulation and the incorporation of biologic response modifiers, such as cytokines or lymphokines, are 2 approaches associated with a reasonable possibility of success. Second, improved methods of radiation enhancement must also be developed. It appears that the improved local control of cancer in the pelvis among patients with rectal cancer can translate into a clinically significant improvement in disease-free survival. Therefore studies of alternative methods of 5FU administration or development of new radiosensitizers should be pursued with vigor.

References

1. Poon MA, O'Connell MJ, Wieand HS, et al. Biochemical modulation of fluorouracil: evidence of significant improvement of survival and quality of life in patients with advanced colorectal carcinoma. J Clin Oncol 1989;7:1407–18.
2. O'Connell M, Maillard J, Martin J, et al (Mayo Clinic and North Central Cancer Treatment Group). A controlled trial of regional intra-arterial FUDR versus systemic 5FU for the treatment of metastatic colorectal cancer confined to the liver. Proc ASCO 1989;8:98.
3. Kemeny N, Daly R, Reichman B, et al. Intrahepatic or systemic infusion of fluorodeoxyuridine in patients with liver metastases from colorectal carcinoma: A randomized trial. Ann Intern Med 1987;107:459–65.
4. Hohn DC, Stagg RJ, Friedman MA, et al. A randomized trial of continuous intravenous versus hepatic intra-arterial floxuridine in patients with colorectal cancer metastatic to the liver: The Northern California Oncology Group Trial. J Clin Oncol 1989;7:1646–54.
5. Chang AE, Schneider PD, Sugarbaker PH, et al. A prospective randomized trial of regional versus systemic continuous 5-fluorodeoxyuridine chemotherapy in the treatment of colorectal liver metastases. Ann Surg 1987;206:685–93.
6. Martin JK Jr, O'Connell MJ, Wieand IIS, et al. Intra-arterial FUdR versus systemic 5FU for hepatic metastases from colorectal cancer. A randomized trial. Arch Surg. (In press)
7. Taylor I, Machin D, Mullee M, et al. A randomized controlled trial of adjuvant portal vein cytotoxic perfusion in colorectal cancer. Br J Surg 1985;72:359–63.
8. Beart R, Moertel C, Wieand H, et al. A randomized trial of 5-fluorouracil (5-FU) by portal vein infusion as surgical adjuvant therapy for colorectal cancer. Society of Surgical Oncology, 1989.
9. Laurie JA, Moertel CG, Fleming TR, et al. Surgical adjuvant therapy of large-bowel carcinoma: An evaluation of levamisole and the combination of levamisole and fluorouracil. J Clin Oncol 1989;7:1447–56.
10. Moertel CG, Fleming TR, MacDonald JS, et al. Effective surgical adjuvant therapy of colon carcinoma: An intergroup study. N Engl J Med 1990;322:352–8.
11. Gastrointestinal Tumor Study Group. Prolongation of the disease-free interval in surgically resected rectal cancer. N Engl J Med 1985;312:1465–72.
12. Gastrointestinal Tumor Study Group. Survival after postoperative combination treatment of rectal cancer. N Engl J Med 1986;315:1294–5.
13. Krook J, Moertel C, Wieand H, et al. Radiation vs. sequential chemotherapy-radiation-chemotherapy. A study of the North Central Cancer Treatment Group and Mayo Clinic. Proc ASCO 1986;5:32.

Discussion

Chairperson: **Minoru Kurihara**

Dr Shigeaki Yoshida (National Cancer Center, Tokyo): I have 2 questions. My first is, what do you think about the possibility of treatment for colorectal cancer with 5FUdR + LV by systemic administration?

Dr O'Connell: That is a good point; the use of a different fluorinated pyrimidine other than 5FU combined with LV. In fact, we are interested in pursuing this very approach, because 5FUdR may be a more selective inhibitor of TS compared to 5FU. Therefore, if the primary rationale of the use of LV as a modulating agent is to enhance the inhibition of TS, perhaps 5FUdR would be a better fluorinated pyrimidine to give in combination. We are planning pilot studies with combinations of 5FUdR + LV since we also feel that this would be a potential strategy to improve further the biochemical modulation of the fluorinated pyrimidines with LV. I do not have any clinical data at this time.

Dr Yoshida: My second question is: in Japan, even patients with colorectal cancer without symptoms are usually indicated to chemotherapy. Would you comment on this?

Dr O'Connell: The question has to do with the patient who has incurable disease. You may have diffuse metastatic disease within the liver and lung, for example, but the patient is feeling well and able to carry on his normal work activities. It has been our philosophy to watch carefully those patients, without initiating chemotherapy until the patient develops either of 2 criteria: a definite sign of tumor growth or significant symptoms related to the cancer process. The reason that this has been our treatment strategy is that a substantial proportion of patients with colorectal cancer have indolent disease that may exist for a period of months and occasionally for a period of years, even without specific treatment. For example, the median time to symptomatic progression in patients with asymptomatic metastatic colorectal cancer is approximately 5–6 months and 20% of patients would still be completely symptom free, 1 year after diagnosis of unresectable metastatic disease. In this group of patients we have elected to study various biologic therapies to see whether we could slow the rate of growth or progression and we have examined BCG, the methanol extraction residue of

BCG, high-dose vitamin C, and, most recently, a somatostatin analog, which is our current study in progress. I would say, though, that if one elects a conservative treatment option of observing these patients without therapy, very close follow-up is indicated, because if one waits too long for the malignant disease to progress to the point where there is malnutrition or significant decrease in performance status, there may be a much lower chance of therapeutic benefit, a lower response rate, and higher toxicity. So in summary, our feeling in this area is that there is a therapeutic window in time when the patient may derive the most benefit from treatment.

Dr Toshifusa Nakajima (Cancer Institute Hospital, Toyko): As I am a surgeon, I am interested in the control of liver metastases, which is also the main prognostic factor in gastric cancer. What do you expect in the way of results with 5FU + LV combination chemotherapy in an adjuvant setting?

Dr O'Connell: We do have experience with 5FU + LV in the treatment of patients with colorectal liver metastases. With systemic administration we have seen an objective response, at least a 50% reduction in tumor size, in 53% of our patients with colon cancer metastatic to liver. It is interesting that we have actually seen higher response rates for tumors within the liver with systemic treatment than we have for tumors in the lung, but I do not understand the reason for this selective response. With regard to adjuvant treatment, we have no data yet. We have, as I indicated, over 350 patients in the national intergroup randomized trial which is comparing the use of 5FU + LV compared to controls, but we have no data at this point. Perhaps another comment here is, in the patient where you, as the surgeon, can remove a metastatic focus from the liver, which occurs in about 5% of patients with metastatic colorectal cancer to the liver, we have studied whether systemic treatment with 5FU + methyl lomustine would be effective as an adjuvant following hepatic resection. Unfortunately, it did not work and we have no encouragement that we affected the course of those patients with adjuvant therapy following hepatic resection.

Dr Nakajima: My second question is that you have mentioned the superiority of intraarterial chemotherapy over systemic administration with regard to tumor regression of liver metastases, but no difference in survival or prolongation. To improve the survival, what do you think of the idea of combination of intraarterial chemotherapy plus systemic chemotherapy for controlling both hepatic and also extrahepatic lesions?

Dr O'Connell: That is precisely the strategy that we are interested in pursuing in our own practice at this time. We are planning to combine intrahepatic therapy with 5FUdR with systemic treatment using 5FU + LV. The specific strategy that we are planning is to start with systemic treatment to give several cycles, perhaps 2 of 5FU + LV up front. The reason that we would like to do this is to allow patients who have occult chemotherapy-resistant disease outside the liver that is not clinically apparent to make itself known so that we can select patients who have a higher probability of having metastatic disease confined to the liver only. Then we plan to implant surgically a catheter into the hepatic arterial tree. We are not going to use the implantable infusion pump device that I mentioned earlier. Rather we will implant an infusion port beneath the skin and use an ambulatory infusion pump to access this, for cost reasons. It is much less expensive to do it by that technique, but I do not recommend this treatment in clinical practice at the moment, because I am concerned that the LV given to modulate 5FU may also modulate the 5FUdR that is given to the liver. Before we will bring this into a major randomized trial we wish to gain experience to know what the appropriate time intervals will be between LV administration and intrahepatic therapy, and what the appropriate doses of 5FUdR will be that can be safely given when there is also LV in the system. However, in summary, we think that a strategy that combines systemic and intraarterial therapy would be a promising one.

Dr Kimitomo Morise (Nagoya University School of Medicine, Nagoya): I would like to ask about the optimal dose of LV in the combination of 5FU + LV. Is 20 mg/m^2 of LV the optimal dose and could you tell me why you did not select a dose of 10 mg/m^2 or 30 mg/m^2?

Dr. O'Connell: I do not know what the optimal dose of LV to give in combination with 5FU is to produce the greatest therapeutic effect, but I can give you some background into our thinking. There are basically 2 bodies of experimental evidence on which we have based our clinical trials. The first was of Dr Hakela, Dr Rustum, and others at Roswell Park Memorial Institute, New York. In the animal model systems that they studied, it was necessary to give an amount of LV to produce 20 μM concentration within the culture medium along with 5FU to produce the greatest inhibition of tumor cells. That amount would correspond to a dose of approximately 500 mg/m^2 given to a human being as a 2-h infusion, and that is the rationale for the high-dose weekly regimen that has been developed by the GITSG. On the other hand, there are other experimental data from Dr Moran and associates from the University of Southern California that indicate that in a different model system—cultured leukemia L1210 cells or a number of different human leukemia cell lines—they could produce optimal inhibition of cell growth by modulated 5FU with a LV concentration of only 1 µM. So there are 2 different bodies of experimental evidence that would suggest that perhaps a high dose would be best, or that perhaps a low dose would be sufficient. That was the basis for our randomized trial, where we give 5FU daily for 5 days and we studied the high-dose and low-dose LV with 5FU for administration daily for 5 days. I think our data rather convincingly indicate that the high dose is not necessary, and that you can effectively modulate with the low dose. However, I think that the interaction with 5FU depends very much on the way that 5FU is given.

A study performed by the GITSG indicated that if one only gave 25 mg/m² of LV with a weekly dose of 5FU, there was no improvement compared to 5FU alone. However when they gave a high dose (500 mg/m²) there was a significant improvement in response rate and so, in my view, the amount of LV necessary to modulate 5FU depends on the schedule of 5FU administration. We are currently testing prospectively, comparing the GITSG weekly high-dose regimen with the low-dose intensive course regimen I have already mentioned to see, by means of a randomized trial, which would be best. We currently have about 110 patients randomized on these 2 treatments and we hope to present the results at the 1991 ASCO meeting.

Why did we use 20 mg/m²? It was a dose that we confidently believed would result in a serum level of LV of least 1 µM, the concentration that was effective in Moran's preclinical system. I quite agree, though, that perhaps 10 mg/m² would do the same thing.

Dr Tsuguhiko Izumi (Showa University School of Medicine, Tokyo): Nowadays, great importance is attached to the quality of life after chemotherapy, as well as the antitumor effect and survival. You have emphasized improvement in performance status, weight gain, and disappearance of symptoms. Would you tell us how quality of life is evaluated in the USA?

Dr O'Connell: In the study that I presented, before the patient was entered into the protocol it was necessary to indicate whether the patient had a clear-cut symptom related to the cancer. About half the patients were symptomatic at the time they entered trial. Every time the patient returned for evaluation, the clinician judged whether that symptom had improved, stayed the same, or worsened. The analysis that was presented here was the percentage of patients who had improvement compared to baseline, on at least at one of their posttreatment observations. We performed the same type of analysis for weight gain in comparing any weight gain observed during therapy compared to the baseline, and also improvement in performance status for the group of patients that had some reduction in performance status at the time they entered the study. If you do not have any impairment in performance status, you cannot get better by taking chemotherapy. So each of those factors was evaluated every time the patients came, and that was the basis for the analysis of quality of life. It was an attempt to assess, by those 3 parameters, what the quality of life of the patients would be.

One also has to take into consideration the toxicity from the treatment and balance that against the improvements in the therapeutic parameters. Indeed, one-third of our patients did have significant ulcerative stomatitis which interfered with their quality of life for a period of usually 5–7, but up to 10 days, if it occurred at all.

There are more formal indices of quality of life that have been developed for a more rigorous evaluation, but some of these are rather complex. I think that this an area that is very clinically pertinent for us as clinicians to evaluate the treatment. Are our patients truly benefiting in terms of symptoms and terms of their quality of life? I think that more effective, concise, easy-to-use indices would be needed for future clinical trials. I certainly agree that this is a very important endpoint that we should all be using when we report, in gastrointestinal cancer or other tumor systems, whether any new therapy is truly better than the previous standard.

Dr Yoshihiro Takai (Tohoku University, School of Medicine, Sendai): You showed some benefit of postoperative radiation combined with 5FU, but I think the question of superiority of postoperative radiation and preoperative radiation is still controversial. Do you have any comment on this?

Dr O'Connell: Yes, on the role of preoperative radiation therapy for rectal cancer. Again, as a single modality, radiation therapy, as I understand, can decrease the local tumor failure rate, whether given before or after surgical removal of the rectal cancer. However, I am not aware of any controlled trials that have demonstrated that radiation therapy given alone can increase the long-term survival or cure rates, given pre- or postoperatively. There are some theoretical reasons why preoperative radiation therapy might give some potential advantage. For example, perhaps it would decrease the tendency of tumor cells that might be dislodged or spilled at the time of surgery to implant locally. That is one of the primary rationales for the use of preoperative treatment. It might make the surgical resection easier for some patients by shrinking the tumor. On the other hand, our clinical staging technology at the present time is so insensitive that we are never certain before the surgery is done whether the patient already has occult metastatic disease, in the liver, the peritoneal cavity, or elsewhere. So the patient might be undergoing unnecessary treatment to the pelvis, already having distant metastatic disease. Also, it is very difficult to know the precise stage of the cancer preoperatively and one might be giving unnecessary radiation therapy to patients with early stage, eg, B1-type rectal cancer, that would have an 80–85% chance of cure without any adjuvant treatment at all. So in balance, when we consider the advantages and disadvantages of preoperative radiation therapy, our current thinking is that we prefer to have the precise pathological staging based upon surgical exploration before subjecting a patient to any adjuvant treatment. I would say for the future, though, that if we did have sensitive ways accurately to stage rectal cancer, perhaps the use of monoclonal antibodies with radioisotopes, perhaps with NMR or methodology using future techniques that have not yet been developed, then the combined use of pre- and postoperative radiation therapy would be a scientific question that we would be very interested in addressing.

So our primary indication for preoperative radiation in rectal cancer now is for patients with fixed tumor who are considered clinically to be unresectable, where we do think there is very significant value of radiation therapy, even converting some of these patients to a resectable state. So we do use radiation therapy very aggressively, but not currently as a preoperative adjuvant treatment, for those reasons.

Dr Koro Sakoda (Kagoshima Medical Association Hospital, Kagoshima): Could you tell us the best choice of treatment for local recurrence after rectal cancer had been resected?

Dr O'Connell: Our current approach to this problem is the use of radiation therapy given by external beam technique, combined with 5FU as a radiation dose-modifier, as a radiation sensitizer. In selected patients, namely those whose tumor would be very small and might be amenable to intraoperative radiation therapy, we would then take the patient who has had external beam radiation therapy and 5FU, perform a surgical laparotomy, attempt to resect any remaining residual tumor, and then use an intraoperative electron beam boost to any residual disease that might be left behind. Dr Gunderson from our institution has been interested in this approach and his early results would indicate that perhaps 30–40% of patients treated with that aggressive technique would be free of progressive rectal cancer 4–5 years from the beginning of therapy, which compared to our historical experience is much better (only 5–10% of patients would be disease free). However, that is an uncontrolled experience and at the present time the Radiation Therapy Oncology Group (RTOG) in the USA is planning a randomized trial which will use external beam radiation therapy plus 5FU versus the same external beam treatment plus 5FU with an intraoperative electron beam boost. That is a scientific way to evaluate whether the expense and the technical complexities of intraoperative radiation therapy will truly be of benefit. We adopt a very aggressive combined modality approach with radiation/chemotherapy/surgery for recurrent rectal carcinomas.

Cancer chemotherapy

Evolving concepts in cancer chemotherapy: Application to intraperitoneal therapy

Franco M. Muggia

University of Southern California Comprehensive Cancer Center, Los Angeles, California

Introduction

For the treatment of solid tumors I believe one needs to optimize chemotherapy and this, in part, means optimizing the local regional intensity of treatment. Such regional enhancement is one of the evolving concepts of optimizing chemotherapy, especially for solid tumors where intrinsic drug resistance is great. A number of ways can be used for intensifying chemotherapy regionally, but here I will focus primarily on intraperitoneal and intracavitary drug treatments. There is, however, also much interest in the intraarterial administration of drugs by various means (infusion or perfusion with flow arrest), especially in the treatment of liver metastases or prime hepatocellular cancer. Other locoregional intensification measures include intrathecal or intraventricular administration, intravesicular and intratumoral methods, and extracorporeal administration, for example, phototherapy.

There are several reasons why drugs should be applied regionally. One is the frequency of local manifestations of tumors that are not amenable to surgical resection. This may be because they involve widespread small tumors that may be resistant to the normal doses of radiation therapy that can be given, especially to the abdomen. Second, there may be pharmacologic sanctuaries, perhaps within serosal cavities, that are not treated well by systemic therapies. The third rationale is that a much higher concentration of drugs can be achieved in the peritoneal cavity, and, therefore, presumably in tumor-bearing areas. Fourth, it may be possible at these concentrations to exploit some interactions between drugs and local measures, such as hyperthermia, and certainly to utilize drug-drug interactions. The fifth reason in favor of such therapy is that if the drug is given within the peritoneal cavity, systemic toxicity can be minimized by simultaneous protective measures applied systemically.

Intraperitoneal therapy provides the rationale for treatment of ovarian cancer

111

and this is the specific example I will discuss. I will describe some of the techniques and concepts of intraperitoneal therapy, introduce the idea of pharmacologic advantage in the context of a phase I study done on the fluoropyrimidine, floxuridine (FUdR). I will then review the data with cisplatin and the platinum analogue carboplatin, with the recognition that so far one cannot conclude whether or not these treatments have led to an overall improvement of results in ovarian cancer. Although I will primarily review treatment in ovarian cancer, these concepts are equally applicable to early stages of gastrointestinal cancer with intraperitoneal spread after resection.

Intraperitoneal therapy in ovarian cancer

The rationale for using intraperitoneal therapy in ovarian cancer is that intraperitoneal spread is a common feature at presentation of this disease. During the course of the disease, detectable metastases outside the peritoneum are unusual until late, except perhaps for pleural manifestations, which occur in 20% of patients. The lethal events in this disease are mostly related to intraperitoneal spread, usually resulting in bowel obstruction. Also, in ovarian cancer, as in many other malignancies of solid tumors especially in gastrointestinal cancer, salvage systemic chemotherapy has been generally ineffective.

Repeated intracavitary drug delivery is now possible, although there are administration problems. The method that we use for intraperitoneal drug delivery is the Port.A.Cath system which has a Tenckhoff catheter in the cavity with a cuff at the peritoneal surface to prevent the entry of infection and which is inserted into a reservoir implanted subcutaneously (Fig 1). It is also possible to have only a Tenckhoff catheter with part of the catheter coming out of the skin, but it requires greater care on the part of the patient. The advantage of the Tenckhoff is that it can be removed without additional surgery, whereas removal of the Port.A.Cath reservoir requires a minor surgical procedure.

Another basic technical concept, introduced by Dedrick and coworkers in the late 1970s at the US National Cancer Institute (NCI), is that of high-volume administration [1]. In the early days of intraperitoneal therapy, administration of a small amount of drug was attempted, but it would not diffuse evenly. The idea of administering at least 2 L of fluid resulted in an even distribution of drug throughout the peritoneal cavity. Other technical aspects of this therapy involve checking that the drug distribution is satisfactory by means of a scan by computed tomography (CT). For this the patient receives intraperitoneal administration of fluid, either Hypaque or Renografin, and the distribution is then assessed to see that it reaches all potential areas of the cavity (over and under the liver, below the left diaphragm, the lesser omental sac, and right and left pelvic gutters and the true pelvis). We recommend that this study be done at the beginning of treatment in those patients who have this implantable peritoneal catheter. This is because such a CT scan can possibly reveal unforeseen problems. For example,

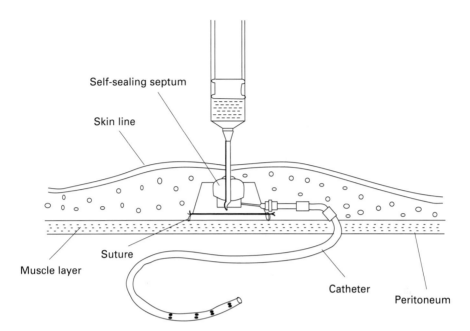

Fig 1   Port.A.Cath intraperitoneal system.

we have seen a patient with ovarian cancer who had a pelvic collection of fluid revealed during CT scanning with contrast. We verified with a needle collection that there were malignant cells in this fluid. The patient had to undergo surgery and dismantling of adhesions between the sigmoid colon and the pelvic side wall with repositioning of the catheter, so that this area was now being treated. This particular patient has survived without manifestations of disease 4 years after intraperitoneal treatment for ovarian cancer and I think that without repositioning the catheter we would not have been successful.

Problems of intraperitoneal therapy

What are some of the problems of intraperitoneal therapy? An obvious problem is that of local drug toxicity. There are some drugs that are notorious for producing peritonitis or sclerosis and are not suitable for repeated administration. One may question how important repeated administration is, but with a drug such as cisplatin, repeated administration is probably important in the treatment of ovarian cancer. The other obvious problem, and I believe that this is the most difficult to overcome in terms of achieving an advantage through intraperitoneal administration, is the uneven drug distribution related to adhesions. Another important problem is that of bulk disease. If the tumor is greater than 2 cm in diameter there is likely to be poor penetration by the drug and the advantage of

113

the intraperitoneal route is totally negated. Therefore the treatment is primarily directed to low-volume disease throughout the peritoneal cavity. This is not uncommon in ovarian cancer and in some of the early stages of gastrointestinal cancer before you detect diffuse metastases.

Finally there are a number of catheter failures and catheter-related complications. With the implantable catheter we do not see infections as readily, in fact they have become quite uncommon. However, problems with outflow are commonly seen; in other words, one can put in a drug, but one cannot take fluid out of the cavity with the catheter functioning as a one-way valve. There are also occasional failures where there is complete occlusion of the catheter, the fluid can at times be administered subcutaneously by error, and perforations into viscera have also been reported. The existence of these problems makes it imperative that the team using intraperitoneal therapy develops a certain experience with its administration technique.

Intracavitary techniques

There are a number of innovations that have been considered in these new approaches to intracavitary therapy. One I mentioned above is the use of large volumes and intermittent dosing, which we feel is important in therapeutic applications in ovarian cancer. Initially when antimetabolites were given, such as methotrexate or fluorouracil (5FU), the group at NCI modelled pharmacologically the administration of timed dwells repeated every 4 h [2]. Unfortunately, this is not a practical procedure because of the problems that develop with outflow and it is also very demanding on the patient. Some groups have advocated continuous intracavitary infusion. There are also some theoretical problems with this since one does not know that the distribution of the drug throughout the cavity will be uniform. It is also a very difficult treatment to carry out in many patients.

We have recently become interested in the combination of hyperthermia with intraperitoneal administration. There is currently also much interest in the use of special carriers such as liposomes, monoclonal antibodies, and radioimmunoconjugates.

Another technique to improve the efficacy of intracavitary therapy involves the concept of systemic neutralization, which has been advanced primarily by Howell et al, at the University of California [3]. If thiosulfate is given intravenously while cisplatin is administered into the peritoneal cavity, one can actually administer larger doses of the cisplatin than would be tolerated under normal circumstances. This is because although a small amount of the neutralizing agent diffuses into the peritoneal cavity, the major aspect of neutralization occurs by rapid excretion of the compound by the kidney, where it ties up and neutralizes cisplatin in the renal tubules. One can therefore give 200 mg/mm^2 of cisplatin

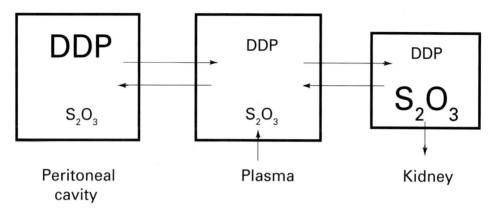

Fig 2 Compartmental model of the current hypothesis showing how thiosulfate serves as a cisplatin (DDP)-neutralizing agent. Reprinted, with permission, from Howell SB et al [3].

intraperitoneally with little renal toxicity. One then has both a very high local effect plus an advantage systemically (Fig 2) [3].

Pharmacological advantages of intraperitoneal therapy

Floxuridine

We performed a study at New York University and the University of Southern California with FUdR (5-fluoro-2'-deoxyuridine, 5FU deoxyriboside). This drug is preferentially used for intraarterial administration because of its greater solubility. It also has a different clearance by the liver than 5FU and therefore may have an advantage in peritoneal administration. It is also the more proximal metabolite of the active nucleotide fluorodeoxyuridylate, which then forms a ternary complex with reduced folates and the enzyme thymidylate synthetase. This particular compound has been shown to synergize more with tetrahydro-folate than would 5FU and there is now a great deal of interest in the administration of leucovorin for the purpose of enhancing the action of fluoropyrimidines (Fig 3) [4]. Finally, it is also substantially more potent on a molar basis than 5FU in its cytotoxicity. Conversely, 5FU in intraperitoneal studies, perhaps related to its basic pH, is more toxic to the peritoneal surfaces and, in fact, its administration may be associated with abdominal pain.

For all these reasons we thought it would be worthwhile investigating whether this particular fluoropyrimidine had advantages over 5FU in intraperitoneal administration. This study was carried out in collaboration with colleagues at both New York University and the University of Southern California.

In the phase I study we began with 500 mg of fluorodeoxyuridine in 2 L of normal saline with 4 mmol/L potassium given on day 1. This was instilled over

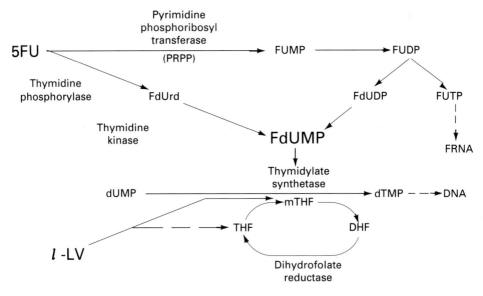

Fig 3 Metabolic pathways of 5FU with the site of *l*-leucovorin (LV) interaction with thymidylate synthetase and FdUMP, once it has been activated to 5,10-methylene tetrahydrofolate (mTHF).

20–30 min and initially we were draining in 4 h. This was eventually found to be unnecessary and we escalated the treatment to 3 consecutive days. Initially we were cautious because fluorodeoxyuridine has a marked time-dependence action, which means that at very low doses over prolonged periods it is more toxic than on a high-dose intermittent schedule. For practical reasons we did not exceed more than 3 days consecutively. The dose escalations were as follows: at 500 mg × 1 we entered 4 patients and then all of them were increased to 1000 mg and

Table 1 Treatment schedule of phase I intraperitoneal FUdR trial.

1. FUdR 500 mg in 2 L of NS with 4 mEq/L KCl on day 1
2. FUdR instilled ip over a 20–30 min period and drained (if possible) after a 4-h dwell time
3. Patients treated every 3–4 wk
4. Dose escalation:

FUdR (mg)	Day	No. of patients
500	1	2
1000	1	2
1000	1,2	2
1000	1,2,3	3
2000	1,2,3	3
3000	1,2,3	3
4000	1,2,3	3

then to 1000 mg × 2. Eventually we reached 3000 mg × 3 days (we did not administer doses per m^2 as we felt that the concentration in the abdomen needed to be fixed and that there should be no major systemic effect of the drug) (Table 1). We have now treated 12 patients with this dose at entry and have shown no systemic effects other than nausea and vomiting occurring a few hours after administration. At 4000 mg and 5000 mg there was one instance each of severe hematologic toxicity.

Pharmacokinetic parameters were obtained in the 7 patients at different doses between 1000 mg and 4000 mg, as shown by the graph in Fig 4. The area under the curve (AUC, the concentration × time in the peritoneal fluid [g/mL/min]) varied from 50 000 to 200 000, whereas in the plasma it varied between 5 and 51. The ratios of peritoneal fluid to plasma FUdR varied from 641 to 8000. It

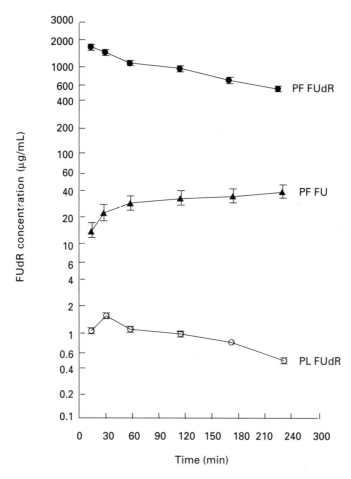

Fig 4 Pharmacokinetics of FUdR 5000 mg in one patient. PF, peritoneal fluid concentration; PL, plasma concentration [Muggia F, Chan K, unpublished].

117

should be emphasized that this is a 3-log advantage: these were staggering concentrations of FUdR over 6 h in the intraperitoneal fluid. It is also significant that there was substantial peritoneal 5FU. So the parent drug (FUdR) can be degraded to 5FU, and is also activated to the nucleotide.

This study thus established the clinical tolerance of a daily × 3 schedule. FUdR was well tolerated, with no evidence of abdominal pain, except in patients who were treated a few days after laparotomy, in which case it appeared to be the distension causing pain, not the drug. Nausea and vomiting were the only notable toxic symptoms. We are currently carrying out a phase II study in ovarian cancer with this drug and about 15 patients have so far entered the trial. So far, the results of tolerance of the drug are being confirmed.

We have also concluded that FUdR is an attractive drug for intraperitoneal administration in combination with other drugs, in particular, leucovorin. We are currently carrying out a phase I pharmacologic study of increasing intraperitoneal doses of leucovorin (80 mg at present) together with intraperitoneal FUdR. It is also being investigated in combination with intraperitoneal cisplatin. A pilot study utilizing both these drugs is being carried out in gastric cancer after resection.

Cisplatin, carboplatin, melphalan, etoposide

Many other drugs have been studied by the intraperitoneal route, primarily in phase I and pharmacologic studies [5]. Although substantial pharmacologic advantage may be confirmed, and for most other drugs a substantial advantage has also been confirmed (with the exception of thiotepa where there is only a 4-fold advantage), it is difficult to predict what the role of intraperitoneal administration will be in clinical oncology (Table 2).

One exception may be cisplatin. At least 3 studies have been carried out with cisplatin at San Diego, the Netherlands Cancer Institute, and Mount Sinai [6,7] with thiosulfate neutralization in the case of 2 of the studies. The ratio of intraperitoneal to plasma concentration is not as great as with some other drugs. However, the drug is more effective against ovarian cancer and produces no marked sclerosis. Therefore cisplatin may be the drug of choice against ovarian cancer by the intraperitoneal route. With carboplatin, the pharmacologic advantage is slightly less than cisplatin, with a suggestion from the Netherlands studies of a lesser penetrance into tumors than cisplatin. However, results from New York University are encouraging in patients with ovarian cancer treated with intraperitoneal carboplatin [8].

Mitomycin C has been used in pharmacologic studies. It is limited for repeated administration by peritonitis, although there is other postoperative experience where this problem has not been encountered. It does have substantial pharmacologic advantages by the peritoneal route.

Melphalan has recently been studied at the Institute Bordet in Belgium by Dr Piccart and in San Diego [9]. It has a good pharmacologic advantage and is of

Table 2 Drugs commonly used in ip drug therapy.

Drug	Institution	Comment	AUC ip plasma
Thiotepa	Montefiore	No advantage to iv	4.3
Cisplatin	UCSD, NKI, Mount Sinai (NY)	Thiosulfate neutralization	12–16
Carboplatin	NKI, NYU, NCOG	? Less penetrance	17
Mitomycin	Leiden, UAz	Peritonitis	32
Melphalan	UCSD, Bordet	+ Glutaminase modulation	57
Etoposide	Fox Chase, UCSD	Protein binding	65
Doxorubicin	NCI	Peritonitis	400
Bleomycin	UAz	Also intrapleural	408
Cytarabine	UCSD	Systemic deamination	474
5FU	NCI, GOG	Saturation kinetics	367
FUdR	USC/NYU	± Leucovorin	640–3000
Mitoxantrone	UAz, MSK, NKI	Peritonitis	1408

UCSD, University of California-San Diego; NKI, Netherlands Cancer Institute; NYU, New York University; NCOG, Northern California Oncology Group; UAz, University of Arizona; NCI, National Cancer Institute; GOG, Gynecology Oncology Group; MSK, Memorial Sloan-Kettering Hospital.

interest in the treatment of ovarian cancer due to the possibility of substituting it for cyclophosphamide, for which there is no rationale for giving intraperitoneally since it needs to be activated by the liver. Therefore, combinations of melphalan and cisplatin would be of interest for future phase III studies. Melphalan has also been modulated in the past by concomitant administration of the enzyme glutaminase, which can lead to depletion of competitive amino acids and may increase the absorption of melphalan by cells in the peritoneal cavity.

Etoposide has been studied at Fox Chase and San Diego [9] with the aim of utilizing the protein binding characteristics of this compound. In the blood the drug is protein bound and is therefore mostly inactive. In the peritoneal cavity, most of the drug is in the free form because of the lesser amounts of protein binding and, therefore, in the active form. So high AUCs may be obtained for both free etoposide and teniposide (which a French group has tested [9]) which has even greater protein binding. This results in an even greater pharmacologic advantage by the intraperitoneal route.

Other drugs

Several other drugs have markedly higher advantages, including the above-cited FUdR. 5FU also has a substantial advantage, though lower than that of FUdR. It demonstrates, as FUdR does, saturation kinetics. A number of the antitumor antibiotics have substantial pharmacokinetic advantages. Unfortunately, doxorubicin causes peritonitis and cannot be used for repeated administration. Bleomycin has aroused interest, primarily for intrapleural use and it also has a considerable pharmacokinetic advantage. The antimetabolite cytarabine has an advantage that relates to its significant deamination when it enters the bloodstream.

Recently there has been interest in the results with mitoxantrone in a clonogenic assay against certain solid tumor cell lines [10]. This drug is extremely potent against solid tumors and it can also be given intraperitoneally in doses leading to a large pharmacologic advantage. Unfortunately, the use of mitoxantrone is also complicated by the development of peritonitis, although not as severe as that associated with doxorubicin. This drug is also being tested by the South West Oncology Group (SWOG) in a phase I study, randomized with FUdR, and the results are awaited with great interest (SWOG, unpublished).

Salvage treatment for ovarian cancer

Table 3 [7] summarizes the results of the Mount Sinai and Netherlands studies in ovarian cancer, which were verified by 3rd-look laparotomies. The laparotomy results showed that intraperitoneal cisplatin led to a negative laparotomy in about one third of the patients, leading to considerable initial enthusiasm. However, a recent update of these results has shown that there are late recurrences in tumors and this indicates that laparotomy cannot be used as a valid or practical endpoint for such studies. We must therefore seek alternative endpoints for clinical trials in intraperitoneal therapy.

Table 3   Results of intraperitoneal cisplatin in ovarian cancer. Reprinted, with permission, from Ozols R [6].

	Mount Sinai	Netherlands Cancer Institute
Patient eligibility	Small-volume disease after induction chemotherapy	
No. of patients	23	21
Cisplatin dose	50 mg/m^2 in 2 L every 3 wk	60–150 mg/m^2 in 2 L every 2–3 wk
No. of cycles	6	6–10
Sodium thiosulfate	Not used	If toxicity developed in previous cycle
Catheter	Temporary catheter in 75% of patients	Tenckhoff
Results	6/19 (32%) negative laparotomy	7/21 (33%) negative laparotomy

Techniques used in these studies also varied. One utilized the Tenckhoff catheter and the other a temporary catheter. The Mount Sinai group did not utilize thiosulfate and therefore the dose of cisplatin was considerably lower (50 mg/m^2). The Netherlands study started at 80 mg/m^2 and escalated, with thiosulfate added for protection if toxicity developed. All these patients had small-volume disease after induction chemotherapy, which was also the criteria for eligibility for the SWOG. The patients had to have small-volume disease, ie, less than 2 cm residual disease at the time of 2nd-look laparotomy.

The San Diego group did not do laparotomies, but they published survival curves which stand as the most encouraging results in salvage chemotherapy (Fig 5). A remarkable 70% survival at 4 years was seen in 25 patients with minimal residual disease treated intraperitoneally with a variety of cisplatin regimens, including cisplatin alone and combinations with cytarabine and bleomycin or doxorubicin in sequential studies [11]. Our results with carboplatin have been only slightly inferior to these and compared favorably with the results of radiation therapy in these circumstances: persistence of disease after chemotherapy, inferior to radiation therapy frontline. The patients with bulky disease, ie, more than 2 cm, however, relapsed quickly. This intraperitoneal route is probably not useful for salvage chemotherapy in these patients, although it is possible that the cisplatin did result in improvement through systemic absorption, but there were no long-term survivors.

Our intraperitoneal carboplatin trial was updated in a study by Speyer [8] of 24 patients, 22 with minimal disease, the other 2 had bulky disease. All patients had had prior cisplatin and 12 had received intraperitoneal cisplatin so that these

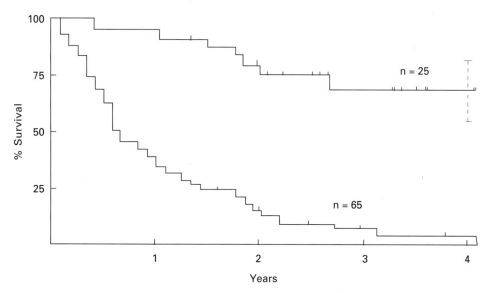

Fig 5   Survival of patients in cisplatin-based ip trials. Top line, patients with small-volume disease; bottom line, patients with bulky disease. Reprinted, with permission, from Howell SD et al [11].

were very heavily pretreated patients. The mean dose of cisplatin for all 24 patients was 560 mg/m^2. Many of these patients came from our frontline treatment with intraperitoneal cisplatin. The toxicity of carboplatin is, unlike cisplatin, primarily hematologic and significantly low platelet nadirs were achieved in a dose escalation scheme. Patients with a creatinine clearance greater than 60 cc/min were escalated preferentially, since they encountered only mild toxicity at lower doses. The patients with very abnormal creatinine clearances from previous cisplatin tolerated no higher than 200 mg/m^2. Escalation in all these patients except one caused severe thrombocytopenia, which limited the further escalation of carboplatin. The therapeutic results, however, were encouraging, with 6 pathologic complete remissions. As in the previous experience with cisplatin, relapses from complete remission occurred, but 3 patients continued free of disease. Six others not subjected to laparotomy have not relapsed up to 39 months after starting carboplatin. Five have progressed after clinical complete remission with the overall median survival exceeding 20 months.

Intraperitoneal treatment as first-line therapy

The efficacy of cisplatin and carboplatin encouraged us to investigate the possibility of using intraperitoneal chemotherapy as the first approach to the treatment of ovarian cancer. From 1979 to 1984 at New York University we combined cisplatin with cyclophosphamide in an intensive fashion [12]. The rationale was to maximize the dose intensity of cisplatin and for that reason we deleted doxorubicin from the primary combination. We believe that there was improved tolerance to a daily × 5 cisplatin schedule, so we used 20 mg/m^2 × 5. Cyclophosphamide 600 mg/m^2 could be given with minimal overlapping toxicity. We assumed that the maximum response would occur within 6 months, as other studies with cisplatin had indicated [13]. In the 2nd study we utilized the same induction schedule, intravenous cisplatin and cyclophosphamide every 21 days, but in this particular study we initially gave 2–4 cycles and then we evaluated further for intraperitoneal therapy, giving cisplatin at 60 mg/m^2 for 3–6 cycles and then a 2nd-look laparotomy. We reasoned that with 52 patients treated in the 1st study and a median survival of 3 years, we could improve this by adding intraperitoneal administration.

Unfortunately the results of this study did not show any definite improvement. However, from it we learned more about the problems and benefits of this type of intraperitoneal therapy. Seventy-five consecutive patients were entered, 7 of whom were stage IV. Most had stage III ovarian cancer and had high grades of disease. About 50% of the patients had substantial amounts of residual disease after laparotomy, although a few had no residual disease and 37% had minimal residual disease. Of the 75 patients entered, we currently have 57 alive, so this is a preliminary report. There are 24 who have so far gone through to surgical verification and have no evidence of disease after completing treatment. Eleven

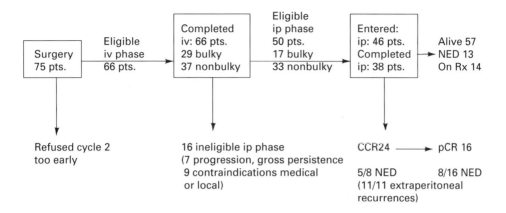

Fig 6   First-line intravenous/intraperitoneal study (New York University): flow of patients.

have relapsed (Fig 6). It is noteworthy that all relapses were extraperitoneal. This indicates that our treatment is actually effective in the peritoneal cavity, but that the dosages that we administered to these patients were ineffective systemically. Therefore the systemic component of the treatment needs to be built up. The other aspect to note is that, of the 75 patients, only 66 were eligible for the intravenous phase; some were ineligible because they refused further therapy or were too early at that point. Of the patients that completed the intravenous phase, only 50 became eligible for the intraperitoneal phase and most of those were nonbulky patients. The reason that the others were not eligible was progression of the disease, growth persistence, or medical or local contraindications such as extensive adhesions for intraperitoneal placement of the catheter.

In summary, we found 2 major problems in this study. First, there were extraperitoneal recurrences and second, there were many patients with bulky disease who could not go on to the intraperitoneal phase of treatment.

The overall survival curve and number of patients alive at 3 years compared to our original 52 patients are quite similar to when we were using intravenous treatment alone. However these were sequential studies and they cannot be strictly compared. Looking at survival by nonbulky versus bulky disease, the median survival, at least of the nonbulky disease patients was as good and these were the majority of patients proceeding on to intraperitoneal cisplatin.

Randomized studies are required and some are ongoing. There is also a study at Memorial Hospital [14] looking at the same induction plus intraperitoneal cisplatin with etoposide. The San Diego group is conducting a random study comparing intraperitoneal to intravenous cisplatin and etoposide. The South West Oncology group study is investigating cisplatin intraperitoneally and intravenous cyclophosphamide compared to both intravenously. Future studies will probably be also carried out on carboplatin, since this can be given for longer periods and on an outpatient basis without extra hydration, which are remarkable advantages.

Conclusions

In summary, the rationale for intraperitoneal cisplatin in ovarian cancer is as follows: the clinical efficacy and its salvage; the correlation between dose intensity and survival noted in some studies; the correlation between the extent of platinum DNA adducts and responses noted by some studies. The concentration required for 73% inhibition in ovarian cancer specimens include 50 mg/mL × 1 h, a concentration that can be reached by intraperitoneal therapy but not systemically (data from Dr Alberts, University of Arizona) [15].

Finally, some of the potential problems and some of the experimental areas in intraperitoneal therapy should be emphasized. As well as failure of distribution of the drug, there is also misinterpretation or inaccuracy of efficacy endpoints. New endpoints should be sought such as improvement in cytological or marker results or time to treatment failure. Some of the studies have also been complicated by entry of patients unlikely to benefit, ie, those with bulky disease. Some investigators have used inadequate antitumor agents and complex regimens in which one agent is not given optimally. For example, there are many studies with intraperitoneal fluorouracil in one dose which may not be the most effective way. There are also inadequate intraperitoneal devices that lead to complications and the adoption of many of these regimens clinically before the confirmation of beneficial results. Nevertheless, there are interesting experimental modalities for the future both in ovarian and gastrointestinal cancer. Drug combinations intraperitoneally, such as FUdR and leucovorin, or combinations supplemented by intravenous therapy. There is the neutralization concept of Howell et al, biochemical modulation agents such as dipyridamole, buthionine sulfoximine, and leucovorin. There is targeting and many biological response modifiers. Other approaches include hyperthermia and laser therapy plus hematoporphyrin.

Workers in the field of cancer chemotherapy have been increasingly concerned with making a greater impact in the treatment of solid tumors. The early challenges of treating tumors with drugs which led to the concepts of combination chemotherapy have been replaced by an awareness of the difficulties of identifying truly active drugs against most of the common tumors. These problems have continued despite the application of ideas such as dose intensification and the introduction of screens to identify drugs effective against these tumors. The possibilities for biochemical modulation and awareness of drug resistance have added new dimensions in our understanding of cancer chemotherapy. The interest in local regional therapy, exemplified by intraperitoneal treatment, brings together many of these concepts and may have future applications in the treatment of ovarian cancer and early stages of gastrointestinal cancer.

124

References

1. Dedrick RL, Myers CE, Bungay PM, et al. Pharmacokinetic rationale for peritoneal drug administration in the treatment of ovarian cancer. Cancer Treat Rep 1978;62:1–9.
2. Speyer JL, Sugarbaker PH, Collins JM, et al. Portal levels and hepatic clearance of 5-fluorouracil after intraperitoneal administration in man. Cancer Res 1982;41:1916–22.
3. Howell SB, Pfeifle CE, Wung W, et al. Intraperitoneal cisplatin with systemic sodium thiosulfate protection. Ann Intern Med 1982;97:845–51.
4. Mini E, Moroson BA, Bertino JR. Cytotoxicity of floxuridine and 5-fluorouracil in human T-lymphoblast leukemia cells: Enhancement by leucovorin. Cancer Treat Rep 1987;71:381–9.
5. Howell SB. Novel aspects of drug delivery. In: ASCO educational booklet 1989. Chicago: American Society of Clinical Oncology and Bostrom Corporation; 1989.
6. Ozols R. Intraperitoneal chemotherapy in the management of ovarian cancer. Semin Oncol 1985;(suppl 4):75–80.
7. Piccart MJ, Speyer JL, Markman M, et al. Intraperitoneal chemotherapy: technical experience at 5 institutions. Semin Oncol 1985;12(suppl 4):90–6.
8. Speyer JL, Richards D, Beller U, et al. Trials of intraperitoneal carboplatin in patients with refractory ovarian cancer. In: Bunn PA, ed. Carboplatin (JM-8). Current perspectives and future directions. Philadelphia: WB Saunders; 1990:153–62.
9. Presentations at the Third International Conference on Intracavitary Therapy, University of California, San Diego, 1988.
10. Alberts DS, Surwit EA, Peng Y-M, et al. Phase I study of mitoxantrone given to patients by intraperitoneal administration. Cancer Res 1989;48:5874–5.
11. Howell SD, Zimm S, Markman M, et al. Long-term survival of advanced refractory ovarian carcinoma patients with small volume disease treated with intraperitoneal chemotherapy. J Clin Oncol 1987;5:1607–12.
12. Beller U, Speyer J, Colombo N, et al. Firstline intraperitoneal chemotherapy in advanced ovarian adenocarcinoma. Proc ASCO 1987;6:113.
13. Omura G, Blessing J, Ehrlich C, et al. A randomized trial of cyclophosphamide and doxorubicin with or without cisplatin in advanced ovarian cancer: A Gynecologic Oncology Group study. Cancer 1986;57:1725–50.
14. Hakes T, Markman M, Reichman B, et al. Pilot trial of high intensity in cyclophosphamide/cisplatin and IP cisplatin for advanced ovarian cancer. Proc ASCO 1989;8:159.
15. Alberts DS, Young L, Mason NL, et al. In vitro evaluation of anticancer drugs against ovarian cancer at concentrations achievable by intraperitoneal adminstration. Semin Oncol 1985;12(suppl 4):38–42.

Discussion

Chairperson: **Makoto Ogawa**

Dr Kiyoji Kimura (National Nagoya Hospital and Nagoya Memorial Hospital, Nagoya): Intraperitoneal administration of anticancer agents is a commonly used technique, often given in the treatment of peritonitis carcinomatosis associated with gastrointestinal cancer. I would like comment on this.

Although it was not particularly mentioned in Dr Muggia's presentation, we believe that the efficacy of chemotherapy depends on the product of cancer tissue concentration of the agents and the duration of contact between the agents and the cancer cells. With regard to this point, intraperitoneal adminstration of drugs is a useful method for increasing the efficacy of chemotherapy. Dr Muggia has described the use of time-dependent drugs, such as 5FU and its analogues. But what do you think when both the time- and concentration-dependent drugs, such as some of the anthracyclines or the alkylating agents are used in a method different from Dr Muggia's? We often employ them after retention of fluid in the peritoneal cavity. Dr Muggia described starting with a Port.a.Cath catheter before ascites occur. I agree with that.

In our cases, when a chemotherapeutic agent is administered into the peritoneal cavity, the drug concentration increases greatly. Despite the high concentration in the peritoneal cavity, the blood concentration is low, less than one-tenth of that of the peritoneal cavity. Using this method of administration, a high tumor effect might be obtained and side effects might be minimal. However, there is still the problem that peritonitis carcinomatosis might cause adhesion after intraperitoneal administration. So I would like to ask Dr Muggia what he thinks about this.

Dr Muggia: First, I would like to say that some of our experiences with the antimetabolites, particularly cytarabine and, we think, FUdR, have shown that there are indications that if one gives them for a longer period of time the efficacy may be improved, although practical limitations usually shortened the treatment. However, a pilot, phase I study by Dr Howell with cytarabine for 5 consecutive days resulted in 2 patients with prolonged, complete regressions of ovarian cancer which have never relapsed, so there may be a very important time-dependent aspect. With drugs like cisplatin, however, we feel that the effect may be both local and systemic, for, as with the antimetabolites, one is really more concerned with the local effects. Fluorinated pyrimidines, particularly, are quite erratic in their systemic toxicities when you give them by the intraperitoneal route, because of their saturation kinetics in clearance. With cisplatin, however, we feel that the effects are both systemic and intraperitoneal. Regarding the prevention of adhesions, I do not think we have an optimal system for the repeated administration of drugs, but it is clear that some drugs can be given repeatedly over short periods of time, and for several months, without causing much in terms of adhesions, except in close proximity to the catheter. Other drugs elicit substantial reactions and it is likely that these drugs will only be delivered for 1 week to several months. For example, for mitoxantrone we just have amended the protocol to give the drug every 2 weeks in small doses to try and maximize the amount of drug that we give during a period of 6 repeated administrations, because if there is too much time between treatments, the adhesion formation will be prohibitive. So we are beginning to learn the problem of adhesion formation. I think that it is drug dependent and that it is also partly dependent on the system of administration.

Lung cancer

Treatment of small cell and non-small cell lung cancer: Current status and future prospects

Daniel C. Ihde

Clinical Investigations Section, National Cancer Institute, NCI-Navy Medical Oncology Branch, Naval Hospital Bethesda, Bethesda, Maryland

Introduction

To begin, I would like to emphasize that the most hopeful thing that can be said about the treatment of lung cancer in the past 5 years is that in the USA, at least, there are some indications that the death rate due to this tumor is starting to diminish in American men. Unfortunately, that is not yet true in American women and nor is it true in either sex in Japan. We must hope that, with greater attention to elimination of cigarette smoking, this public health scourge, which has now spread from the USA to Asia, can be eliminated.

Small cell lung cancer

Lung cancer is the most common cause of cancer death in both men and women in the USA. It is a major public health problem. If small cell lung cancer, which constitutes 20–25% of all lung cancers in the USA, were considered a separate malignancy, American Cancer Society estimates for 1988 indicate that it would be the 6th most common cancer in terms of number of newly diagnosed cases and the 4th most common cause of cancer death (Table 1).

Small cell lung cancer is distinguished from other cell types of lung cancer by, among other characteristics, its rapidly inexorable clinical course in the absence of treatment and its increased responsiveness to cytotoxic chemotherapy. Prior to the utilization of modern combination chemotherapy in this disease, median survival of patients with localized or limited-stage and more advanced extensive-stage disease was 3 and 1.5 months, respectively. Five-year survival of limited-stage patients subjected to surgical resection or chest radiotherapy was 3% or less. Combination chemotherapy with or without chest irradiation has improved median survival approximately 4–5 fold, with 12–16 months' survival in limited

131

Table 1 Most common cancers in the USA when small cell lung cancer is considered as a separate malignancy (1988 American Cancer Society estimates).

New cases	Deaths
1) Colorectal	1) Non-small cell lung
2) Breast	2) Colorectal
3) Non-small cell lung	3) Breast
4) Prostate	4) Small cell lung
5) Bladder	5) Prostate
6) Small cell lung	6) Pancreas
7) Endometrium	7) Non-Hodgkin lymphoma
8) Non-Hodgkin lymphoma	8) Stomach

and 7–11 months' survival in extensive disease being commonly reported. Five-year survival of 6–12% in limited disease can be anticipated with current optimal treatment, but long-term survival in extensive disease is only anecdotal [1].

Recent therapeutic developments

Unfortunately there has been little discernible improvement in survival of small cell lung cancer patients since the introduction of combination chemotherapy in the late 1970s. Below, I shall discuss recent therapeutic developments, including the introduction of the promising etoposide + cisplatin regimen. I will review the value of chest irradiation, documentation that maintenance chemotherapy yields little or no benefits, and the role of surgical resection of the primary tumor. Finally, I will refer to several experimental treatment approaches that are now being evaluated.

Etoposide/cisplatin

Although etoposide/cisplatin is an active drug combination in several other tumors, including testicular cancer, this regimen was first studied in small cell lung cancer as a salvage program for patients who had failed other chemotherapy. At the University of Toronto, etoposide/cisplatin produced a 42% response rate and 17-week median survival in 42 patients, better results than were seen in 18 contemporaneously treated, similar patients given etoposide alone [2]. This led to the evaluation of this treatment in previously untreated patients. In Toronto 11 patients with limited, and 20 with extensive disease with cardiac, pulmonary, or other organ dysfunction were entered into the study. They received etoposide/cisplatin as their sole chemotherapeutic regimen. The overall and complete response rates, median survival, and 2-year survival [3] were similar to expected results with commonly used 3- and 4-drug regimens in both limited and extensive regimens (Table 2).

Two early clinical trials by Sierocki [4] and Woods [5] employed etoposide/cisplatin as initial chemotherapy for 6 and 12 weeks, respectively, followed by the frequently prescribed chemotherapy program of cyclophosphamide/doxorubicin/vincristine (CAV). No patient among the 38 and 49 who entered these trials showed an improved response status when CAV was given following completion of etoposide/cisplatin. This suggested that residual tumor masses that were present after etoposide/cisplatin therapy contained very few cells that were sensitive to the drugs in CAV.

Table 2 Etoposide/cisplatin as sole chemotherapy for small cell lung cancer patients with organ dysfunction. Reproduced, with permission, from Evans et al [3].

	Limited	Extensive
No. patients	11	20
CR + PR	82%	75%
CR	64%	25%
Median survival	14 mo	10 mo
2-year survival	12%	0%

In contrast to the nonrandomized studies mentioned which did not directly address whether etoposide/cisplatin improves survival in small cell lung cancer, 2 recent randomized trials have indicated that the addition of etoposide/cisplatin to CAV is associated with survival benefits. In a Canadian study by Evans in extensive-stage disease [6], 289 patients received either CAV alone or CAV alternating with etoposide/cisplatin. In a US study in limited-stage disease [7], 148 patients, after completing 6 cycles of CAV, received either 2 cycles of etoposide/cisplatin or no further therapy. In both of these trials, patients who received etoposide/cisplatin in addition to CAV lived significantly longer, although the magnitude of survival benefit was quite modest in the extensive-stage trial. This trial does not, however, answer the question of whether the program alternating CAV and etoposide/cisplatin chemotherapy was superior because of the alternating strategy, as first proposed by Goldie and Coldman, or simply because etoposide/cisplatin is a regimen that is superior to CAV. Early results from 2 large 3-arm studies that attempted to answer this question do not yet conclusively resolve the issue. In each case etoposide/cisplatin, CAV, and alternating treatment with both regimens were compared according to a randomized study design. The Japanese trial [8] included both limited- and extensive-stage patients, while the South Eastern Cancer Study Group [9] administered only 4 cycles of chemotherapy to the patients receiving etoposide/cisplatin and 6 cycles to patients on the other 2 arms. Currently, the Japanese study demonstrates an improved response rate in the 2 arms containing etoposide/cisplatin and improved response duration in the alternating chemotherapy arm. No differences in

133

response rate were observed in the US study. In both trials, patients who failed with CAV and who then received etoposide/cisplatin as their 2nd therapy had higher response rates than patients who failed etoposide/cisplatin and then received CAV. At this time, however, no significant survival differences can be seen in either study. Further follow-up may reveal significant findings. At present etoposide/cisplatin alone and alternating etoposide/cisplatin and CAV, which has the advantage of limiting the total doses of doxorubicin, cisplatin, and vincristine, 3 drugs with important cumulative nonhematologic toxicities, appear to be acceptable therapies for small cell lung cancer.

Etoposide/cisplatin may have the additional advantage of possessing at least the equivalent antitumor activity of other commonly used regimens at doses that produce only mild myelosuppression. In a small randomized study of approximately 70 patients being conducted at the US National Cancer Institute (NCI), standard doses of etoposide/cisplatin (total doses per course of 240 mg/m^2 and 80 mg/m^2, respectively) have produced complete response rates and survival almost identical to a regimen administering 67% higher total doses of 400 mg/m^2 of etoposide and 135 mg/m^2 of cisplatin [10]. Median nadir white cell counts and platelet counts are much higher on the standard dose arm, which therefore possesses a much better therapeutic index than high-dose etoposide/cisplatin. Thus, relatively nontoxic doses of etoposide/cisplatin are a very acceptable program for the treatment of small cell lung cancer.

In summary, etoposide/cisplatin is probably the most commonly used chemotherapy regimen for small cell lung cancer at present in the USA. It is active in some patients who have failed CAV treatment. There is little improvement in response status when CAV is administered after etoposide/cisplatin. In 2 randomized studies using alternating and sequential chemotherapy programs, survival was improved by adding etoposide/cisplatin to CAV. Ongoing randomized trials to evaluate the efficacy of etoposide/cisplatin compared to CAV and its role in alternating chemotherapy programs have not yet established etoposide/cisplatin as the single most effective chemotherapy program in current use. It is, however, a regimen with a very favorable therapeutic index.

Radiotherapy

Because of the high frequency of tumor regression which it induces, chest radiotherapy was the mainstay of therapy for small cell lung cancer in the 1960s. When chemotherapy was found to be highly effective during the 1970s, most physicians continued to administer chest irradiation as part of the treatment program. Good results were obtained in some limited-stage disease studies using chemotherapy alone, and the role of chest irradiation in localized small cell lung cancer began to be questioned. Retrospective data from the literature reviewed in 1980 suggested that chemotherapy with radiotherapy and chemotherapy alone produced equivalent overall response rates, complete response rates, and median survival [11]. It was suggested that 2-year disease-free survival might be superior with the addition of chest irradiation (Table 3). However, only within the past few years have sufficient data become available from randomized trials of chemotherapy with or without thoracic radiotherapy to allow meaningful conclusions to be drawn.

Table 3 Combined modality therapy vs chemotherapy alone in limited small cell lung cancer: retrospective data in 1980.

	No. of patients	CR+PR	CR	Median surv. (mo)	2-yr df surv.
Chemo + RT	492	76%	50%	9–18	17%
Chemo alone	246	81%	52%	10–14	7%

There is little doubt that combined modality therapy is more toxic than chemotherapy alone when treating this tumor. Significantly increased toxicities found with added irradiation in randomized trials include myelosuppression in 3 of 6 studies, pulmonary and esophageal toxicity in 4 of 6, and weight loss in 1 of 2. Various measures of antitumor effectiveness are also often favorably influenced. Combined modality therapy was superior to chemotherapy alone in terms of complete response rate in 3 of 4 randomized studies, of control of the local tumor complex in 5 of 7, and in terms of overall survival assessed by the log rank test in 4 of 7. The relative proportion of 2-year survivors was at least 50% greater with added radiotherapy in 3 of 7 studies [12].

The temporal relationships between the delivery of chemotherapy and radiotherapy may be influential in determining whether a survival advantage of combined modality therapy can be demonstrated. When administration of chemotherapy was not delayed to give irradiation, either by administering both forms of treatment concurrently or simultaneously or by alternating the 2 treatments so rapidly that the interval between chemotherapy cycles was no longer than if irradiation had not been given, survival in most randomized studies was improved. Two of 3 trials with concurrent, and the only randomized trial of alternating chemotherapy, showed improved survival with combined modality treatment. In contrast, when chemotherapy was delayed so that irradiation could be given in isolation, so-called sequential treatment, which has been observed to produce less toxicity, only 1 of 3 randomized studies demonstrated better survival. Thus it appears that the more intensive and toxic methods of combined modality treatment which do not compromise chemotherapy delivery may well be preferred. It should be emphasized, however, that these different temporal methods of combining chemotherapy with radiation have never been directly compared in prospective randomized trials.

Intensive combined modality therapy in limited-stage small cell cancer is usually highly effective in improving local control within the radiotherapy portal. Figure 1 shows the data from the NCI randomized trial [13] displaying actuarial freedom from failure at the site of the primary tumor complex and regional lymph nodes. Although approximately the same number of complete responders to each type of therapy first failed solely in the chest, as shown by the 5 failures in each arm of the graph, the much higher proportion of complete responders with combined modality therapy led to a highly significant improvement in local tumor control when thoracic radiotherapy was added to chemotherapy.

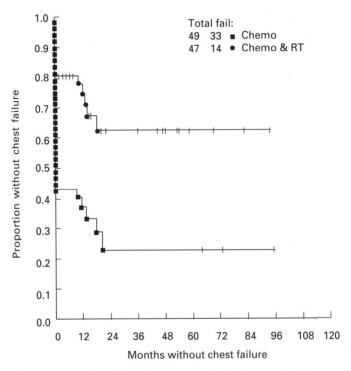

Fig 1   Actuarial freedom from chest failure in patients with limited small cell lung cancer treated with either chemotherapy alone or chemotherapy and radiotherapy (NCI randomized trial). Reprinted, with permission, from Bunn PA et al [13].

Improvements in survival with combined modality therapy, however, are much less impressive than improvements in local control. Reasons for this are illustrated in actuarial survival data from our randomized trial [13] which demonstrate an increase in median survival from 12 to 15 months with the addition of chest irradiation and a 2–4-year survival frequency of 25% with combined modality therapy, compared to 8% with chemotherapy alone (Fig 2). The majority of deaths with both combined modality treatment and chemotherapy alone were due to distant metastatic relapse. In addition, early deaths from pulmonary toxicity on the combined modality arm also reduced the difference in survival

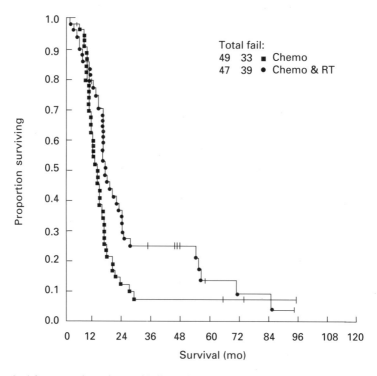

Fig 2 Survival frequency in patients with limited small cell lung cancer treated with either chemotherapy alone or chemotherapy and radiotherapy (NCI randomized trial). Reprinted, with permission, from Bunn PA et al [13].

between the 2 forms of therapy. Finally, only 1 of the 5 late deaths beyond 4 years on the combined modality arm was due to recurrent small cell lung cancer. Three of these deaths were due to development of new second primary lung cancers, almost certainly due to the cigarette smoking that caused the original small cell carcinoma. Thus, in our study, as well as in other randomized trials that showed significant increased survival, this increase was modest, principally due to the failure of available chemotherapy to control micrometastatic disease. So despite the modest but almost certainly real benefits of combined modality therapy, improved systemic treatment still has far greater potential to increase survival in limited small cell lung cancer than do improved forms of local and regional therapy.

What approaches might be utilized to improve the results of combined modality treatment of small cell lung cancer? Clearly the most important would be better systemic therapy that could eradicate occult distant metastases in a greater proportion of patients. This would make overall survival more dependent upon the success of local control, which is very favorably affected by chest irradiation. Other approaches have focused on lessening the toxicity of chemoradiotherapy.

Several groups have now found that etoposide/cisplatin is a chemotherapy regimen that can be given concurrently with irradiation with less pulmonary toxicity than other regimens tested so far. Hyperfractionated irradiation, such as twice-daily radiotherapy, should, in theory, be less toxic to pulmonary tissue and, because of the absence of a shoulder on the radiation survival graph of small cell lung cancer in vitro, might be equally as effective as conventional fractionation against small cell carcinoma tissue. Finally, rapidly alternating split-course chemoradiotherapy appears to be associated with less pulmonary toxicity than concurrent irradiation in uncontrolled data.

In summary, a modest, but real survival gain with addition of chest radiotherapy to chemotherapy has been shown in a majority of randomized clinical trials in limited stage small cell lung cancer. Concurrent or alternating combined modality regimens that do not delay chemotherapy administration to deliver the irradiation appear to be superior. There is definitely increased toxicity with combined modality therapy compared to chemotherapy alone. The regimen with the best therapeutic index is uncertain. Finally, uncontrolled systemic tumor is still the major cause of treatment failure in this disease.

Duration of chemotherapy

When chemotherapy was first utilized in the treatment of small cell lung cancer, most therapeutic regimens administered drugs for at least 2 years in the small fraction of patients who had not developed progressive tumor by that time. Gradually, investigators began to reduce the duration of chemotherapy administration, without obvious compromises in therapeutic outcome. One influential retrospective study of the value of maintenance chemotherapy came from the University of Toronto [14] in the early 1980s (Table 4).

In 2 consecutive trials of the CAV chemotherapy program with chest irradiation in 147 and 320 patients, respectively, the planned duration of chemotherapy in patients who continued to respond to treatment was 61 and 18 weeks. The frequency of patients with limited disease and fully ambulatory performance

Table 4 CAV + radiotherapy with or without maintenance chemotherapy: retrospective comparison. Reproduced, with permission, from Feld R et al [23].

	CAV-1	CAV-2
Duration chemoRx	61 wk	18 wk
No. of patients	147	320
Limited stage	45%	48%
Performance status	88%	86%
Response rate (CR+PR)	83%	84%
Median survival	43 wk	41 wk
2-year survival	8%	8%

status was similar in both studies. Overall response rates, median survival, and 2-year survival were virtually identical in the 2 trials, suggesting the additional 43 weeks of chemotherapy given to the first group of patients was of little benefit.

In the past few years, data from randomized clinical trials addressing the question of the value of continued or maintenance chemotherapy have matured. Results from Australian [5], European [15], and US [16] studies (Table 5) in which patients in various response categories, ranging from complete responders only to all patients without obvious disease progression, were randomized to continue chemotherapy for an additional 7 to 10 cycles or to stop treatment. Both limited- and extensive-stage disease were included in the 2 largest trials. In 2 studies the time to development of progressive disease was significantly increased with maintenance chemotherapy, but in none was there survival advantage to continued chemotherapy. In the very small fraction of patients who are cured by chemotherapy it is self-evident that maintenance chemotherapy beyond the point at which the tumor is eradicated is of no benefit. These trials also suggest, similar to findings in multiple myeloma, a tumor that is never curable with chemotherapy, that continued drug therapy in small cell lung cancer might only prolong the duration of first remission without having any impact on survival.

Table 5 Randomized trials of maintenance chemotherapy in small cell lung cancer.

	Response	Stage	Cycles chemo	No. of patients	Significant difference in:	
					Time to PD	Survival
Woods	CR/PR	LD/ED	4/14	96	No	No
Ettinger	CR	ED	NR	73	Yes	No
Splinter	CR/PR/ NC	LD/ED	5/12	426	Yes	No

LD, limited disease; ED, extensive disease; NR, not reported.

It is obvious that patients who receive protracted chemotherapy have greater treatment-induced toxicity than patients who do not. A less obvious benefit from refraining from administration of maintenance chemotherapy may be that patients with shorter initial duration of chemotherapy, and thus a longer time off drug treatment prior to tumor progression, are more likely to respond to and be palliated by 2nd-line or salvage chemotherapy. Data from 3 phase II trials of etoposide/cisplatin salvage therapy illustrate this point (Table 6). Response rates were over 50% in studies from Toronto and Vanderbilt [17,18], in which initial chemotherapy had a planned duration of 4–5 months, and therefore a median time of 3–5 months off treatment elapsed before the salvage etoposide/cisplatin

Table 6 Etoposide/cisplatin salvage therapy in small cell lung cancer related to duration of prior chemotherapy.

	Prior chemoRx		No. of	Response
	Duration	Time off	patients	rate
Toronto	4.5 mo	3 mo	78	55%
Vanderbilt	5 mo	5 mo	29	52%
NCI (USA)	7 mo	1 mo	29	12%

program was administered. In contrast, our study at the NCI [19] was conducted in patients who had been on continuous chemotherapy with 6 drugs for a median of 7 months and had a median time of only 1 month off treatment before etoposide/cisplatin. In this setting we observed a response rate of only 12%. Similar results have recently been reported from Italy in a trial of 2nd-line therapy for small cell lung cancer with teniposide (VM26). In addition, the increased likelihood of response at the time of relapse to the administration of the chemotherapy regimen that produced the initial response has long been known to be dependent on the interval from discontinuation of initial chemotherapy to relapse in Hodgkin's disease. These results of salvage therapy in small cell lung cancer are entirely consistent with this concept.

In summary, retrospective data suggest little benefit from administration of chemotherapy for more than 3–5 months in responding patients with small cell lung cancer. Recently completed randomized trials support this concept, although maintenance chemotherapy may delay the time to first relapse. Withholding maintenance chemotherapy clearly reduces toxicity, thus increasing the therapeutic index of chemotherapy, and may improve the response to chemotherapy given at relapse. Therefore, discontinuing chemotherapy after 4 to 6 months in patients with complete or partial response is currently recommended.

Surgical resection

There has been a reawakening of interest in surgical resection in small cell lung cancer. After a UK Medical Research Council study showed that chest irradiation led to modestly better survival than attempted surgical resection in patients with apparently operable small cell carcinoma, many thoracic surgeons in North America abandoned operative intervention. However, it was reported in the early 1980s that a small number of patients undergoing more comprehensive preoperative staging procedures could be cured with surgical resection alone. Many groups have reported a superior outcome for patients undergoing surgical resection prior to chemotherapy or chemoradiotherapy compared to other limited-stage patients. There is a high frequency of relapse in the primary site after chemotherapy, even with added irradiation, but the primary tumor is an infrequent site of relapse after surgery. However, on careful literature review, there is no definite survival impact in initially surgically resected patients compared to similar patients who did not undergo surgical resection prior to their chemotherapy. Therefore, several groups have become interested in performing surgical resection of limited-stage small cell cancer only after the initial response to chemotherapy.

The rationale for this approach includes the immediate treatment of occult metastatic disease with chemotherapy and the fact that only chemoresponsive patients, those most likely to benefit, will be subjected to the risk of surgery. In addition, comprehensive initial staging procedures are less often needed when chemotherapy is the initial treatment and, after chemotherapy-induced tumor regression, a larger fraction of patients may be surgical candidates. A review of early uncontrolled studies of this approach [20] reveals the following. There is no excessive postoperative mortality after initial treatment with chemotherapy. No viable tumor is found in 5–20% of resected specimens and these patients, not surprisingly, have better survival. In some patients non-small cell cancer elements predominate in the resected specimen and surgery may well be the best treatment for such patients. Resected patients have a good prognosis with approximately 27% disease-free survival. Initial mediastinal staging has usually not been done in these studies, but some data suggest that patients with pathologically documented mediastinal node involvement have a poor outcome when resection is attempted after chemotherapy response. Finally, there is no obvious marked improvement in survival when all patients beginning chemotherapy, with the intent of operating on responding patients, are considered.

A randomized trial addressing the value of surgical resection after chemotherapy for small cell lung cancer is currently being conducted by the North American Lung Cancer Study Group. Patients are randomized to chemotherapy followed by chest irradiation versus chemotherapy followed by attempted surgical resection and postoperative irradiation. Over 120 patients have been randomized and the initial survival analysis is awaited. The following preliminary conclusions concerning this neoadjuvant chemotherapy approach can be justified.

Surgical resection has been possible in 18–37% of selected patients beginning chemotherapy with intent to operate eventually, possibly a higher fraction at the time of diagnosis. There has been marked variability in patient selection, criteria for operability and resectability, and duration of preoperative chemotherapy in these pilot studies. Resected patients have superior survival to other patients with limited small cell lung cancer, especially if there is no residual viable cancer in the surgical specimen. Current uncontrolled studies are not conclusive regarding survival advantage or definition of subsets of patients who benefit. Therefore, the results of the large randomized Lung Cancer Study Group are awaited and will doubtless be influential in determining the future application of this approach.

Strategies to improve chemotherapy

Several novel strategies for improving the results of chemotherapy are currently under evaluation in clinical trials. Perhaps the most important is the use of investigational agents as initial therapy for carefully selected patients with extensive disease. The Eastern Cooperative Oncology Group has recently demonstrated in a randomized trial that such an approach does not compromise survival even if the investigational drug is inactive, provided standard combination chemotherapy is administered at the first sign of worsening symptoms, nonresponse, or treatment failure. It is to be hoped that vigorous application of this strategy will allow identification of more active chemotherapeutic agents, which are desperately needed in this disease.

Other strategies of interest include the following: administration of hematopoietic growth factors with chemotherapy either to reduce toxicity or to permit dosage escalation and perhaps greater tumor cell kill; short-course weekly chemotherapy, which has given promising results in a few studies; daily oral etoposide, which has demonstrated a higher than expected response rate in previously treated patients; interferon maintenance treatment for responders to chemotherapy, which has shown borderline survival prolongation in one randomized study; and the utilization of chemotherapy alone to induce tumor regression in brain metastases.

Our group has been performing in vitro drug sensitivity testing of cell lines developed from patients entered on a prospective clinical trial, and correlating the results of in vitro drug sensitivity of patients' cell lines with their clinical response to chemotherapy [21]. Table 7 shows the data on the in vitro sensitivity to 7 drugs known to be clinically active against small cell lung cancer in cell

Table 7 Drug sensitivity of cell lines from untreated patients responding and not responding to initial etoposide/cisplatin therapy.

	Response (n=15)	Nonresponse (n=6)	p value
Mean % active* drugs	46%	5%	0.001
Mean % cell survival (all drugs tested)	55%	82%	0.009
Mean % cell survival (3 most active drugs)	34%	70%	0.009
Mean % cell survival (etoposide†)	41%	75%	0.021
Mean % cell survival (cisplatin)	55%	67%	0.43

*Cell survival <50% at reference concentration.
†p also < 0.05 for doxorubicin, vincristine, and mechlorethamine.

lines from our previously untreated patients who either responded or did not respond to 12 weeks of etoposide/cisplatin chemotherapy. Fifteen patients responded and 6 did not. The mean percentage of "active" drugs, defined as cell survival of less than 50% at the reference concentration for each drug in vitro, the mean percent cell survival for all drugs tested, and the mean percent cell survival for etoposide were all significantly different in cell lines from responding and nonresponding patients. The mean percent cell survival for cisplatin was not significantly different in cell lines from the 2 groups. However, the mean percent cell survival for doxorubicin, vincristine, and mechlorethamine were each as closely correlated with clinical response to etoposide/cisplatin as was the mean percent cell survival for etoposide.

These results suggest that in vitro drug sensitivity of cell lines taken directly from patients correlates well with clinical response to chemotherapy in the patients from whom the cell lines were derived. However, since several drugs in addition to etoposide were correlated to clinical response to etoposide/cisplatin, these cell lines appeared to be either generally sensitive or generally resistant to most of the drugs tested. This suggests that in vitro testing of small cell carcinoma cell lines might only be of marginal use in selecting specific chemotherapeutic agents to treat an individual patient. A more productive area of investigation with human cancer cell lines may be to study mechanisms of drug resistance and to screen for new chemotherapeutic agents.

An example of how human cell lines might be used to investigate drug resis-

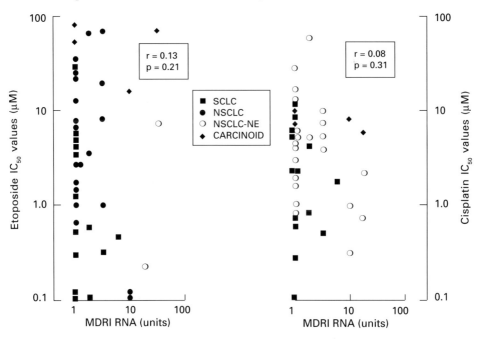

Fig 3 Lack of correlation between *MDR*1 RNA and in vitro chemosensitivity.

tance mechanisms is shown in Fig 3. The graphs display multidrug resistance or (*MDR*1) gene expression, as assessed by messenger RNA levels in over 30 lung cancer cell lines, correlated with in vitro inhibitory concentration 50% (IC_{50}) values for etoposide (on the left) and cisplatin (on the right). It should be noted that cell lines that express the multidrug resistance gene would be expected to be resistant only to etoposide, and not to cisplatin. As is evident there is no significant correlation between the *MDR*1 RNA levels and the IC_{50} values for the cell lines with either etoposide or cisplatin. Furthermore, there was no correlation between *MDR*1 expression and clinical response to chemotherapy or whether or not the cell line was established from a patient who had previously been treated with chemotherapy. These results suggest that *MDR*1 expression is unlikely to be a frequent mechanism for drug resistance in lung cancer [22].

Non-small cell lung cancer

In comparison to small cell lung cancer, patients with non-small cell cancer have less frequent distant metastases at the time of diagnosis, sometimes follow a slower or more indolent course, are more often surgically resectable, less often respond to chest irradiation, are similarly infrequently cured with radiotherapy, and less often respond to cytotoxic chemotherapy. Even though local and regional forms of treatment, especially surgical resection, can cure a much greater fraction of patients with non-small cell than with small cell cancer, the presence of undetected distant metastatic disease is still the major cause of death, even in patients with pathological stage I resected disease who are not cured by surgery.

Data from the Lung Cancer Study Group (Table 8) indicate that approximately two-thirds of first relapses, ie, all relapses except for those in involved lung or the mediastinum, are at distant metastatic sites [23]. Distant metastases are an even more formidable problem in patients with greater bulk of local regional disease. Thus, effective systemic treatment is necessary in order to produce any major improvement in survival of non-small cell cancer and chemotherapy in this disease has so far been ineffective.

Table 8 Site of first relapse in resected stage I non-small cell lung cancer (158 first relapses) (390 patients). Reprinted, with permission, from Feld R et al [23].

Site	%
Involved lung	26
Brain	21
Bone	13
Contralat. lung	13
Mediastinum	7
Other distant site	21
Second 1° lung	4.9

There are several recent positive trials in increasingly more localized stages of non-small cell lung cancer which suggest that chemotherapy may be currently, for the first time, having a biological effect on the disease. It should be noted, however, that for each degree of tumor dissemination, multiple negative clinical studies also exist. Figure 4 shows the survival of 3 groups of patients with disseminated metastatic non-small cell lung cancer randomized to receive vindesine/cisplatin, cyclophosphamide/doxorubicin/cisplatin (CAP), or best supportive care alone in a 3-arm trial carried out by the Canadian National Cancer Institute [24]. Although the magnitude of survival difference was minor, patients on both chemotherapy arms, especially vindesine/cisplatin, lived significantly longer than patients who received supportive care.

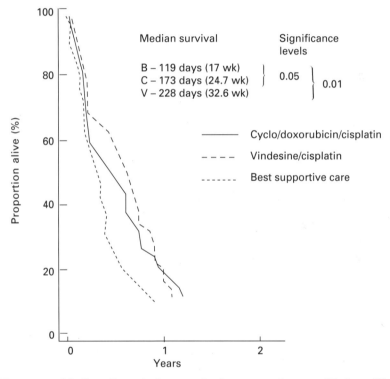

Fig 4   Three arm-trial. Overall survival curves for best supportive care (B) (n = 50), cyclophosphamide/doxorubicin/cisplatin (C) (n = 43), and vindesine/cisplatin (V) (n = 44).

The Cancer and Leukemia Group B recently reported a positive randomized trial, employing 5 weeks of neoadjuvant chemotherapy with vinblastine and cisplatin or no chemotherapy prior to definitive chest irradiation in good prognosis, limited-stage, inoperable patients [25]. In over 150 evaluable patients, median follow-up was 22 months. A significant survival advantage was seen in the chemotherapy-treated patients, whose median survival was almost doubled.

145

At Memorial Sloan-Kettering Cancer Center, a presurgical neoadjuvant chemotherapy pilot study has been performed in patients with ipsilateral mediastinal node enlargement detected by chest X ray [26]. In historical experience at this institution, a 14% resection rate and a 6% 3-year survival in resected patients have been noted in this group. Two to 3 courses of mitomycin C, a vinca alkaloid, and cisplatin in 41 patients produced a 73% response rate, including 17% complete responses. The surgical resection rate was 51%, with over one third of resected specimens not containing cancer. The 3-year survival rate is now 34% in this ongoing study.

The Lung Cancer Study Group performed a randomized trial of postoperative radiation with or without CAP chemotherapy in 164 patients with marginally resectable non-small cell lung cancer [27]. The number of recurrences was significantly reduced and there was a reduction in deaths from cancer and deaths from all causes of borderline statistical significance with the administration of CAP in addition to radiotherapy (Table 9).

Table 9 Recurrence and death rates in 164 patients.

	CAP + RT		RT
No. of patients	78		86
No. of recurrences	50		66
Rate per person per year	0.466		0.838
Mantel-Haenszel (p)		0.004	
Wilcoxon-Gehan (p)		0.001	
No. of deaths from cancer	44		57
Rate per person per year	0.326		0.489
Mantel-Haenszel (p)		0.066	
Wilcoxon-Gehan (p)		0.030	
No. of deaths, all causes	55		64
Rate per person per year	0.408		0.549
Mantel-Haenszel (p)		0.133	
Wilcoxon-Gehan (p)		0.047	

Finally, in the group of patients with presumably the least tumor burden, those who have undergone complete surgical resection with specimen margins pathologically free of cancer, the Lung Cancer Study Group randomized patients to receive CAP chemotherapy or immunotherapy with BCG and levamisole [28]. Once again, disease-free survival was significantly improved (Fig. 5) by chemotherapy that has only extremely modest efficacy in disseminated non-small cell lung cancer, and deaths from cancer and overall death rate were only marginally improved. I think the results of this trial, although there is not an untreated

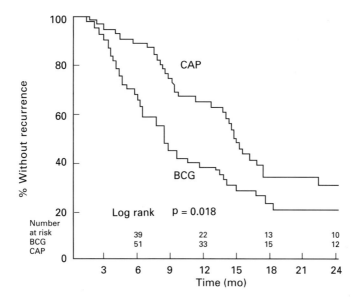

Fig 5 Life-table analysis comparing disease-free interval in a group of lung cancer patients given adjuvant immunotherapy with that in a group given adjuvant chemotherapy.

control arm, are given additional plausibility by the previous study in which chemotherapy also had some effect on disease-free interval.

In my opinion, none of these controlled and uncontrolled clinical trials convincingly demonstrate such a substantial therapeutic effect that any survival improvement in the entire population of patients with non-small cell lung cancer could reasonably be anticipated. Nonetheless, even such marginal chemotherapeutic activity was never noted in non-small cell lung cancer prior to the present decade. These and other results should, I believe, revive interest in clinical investigations evaluating novel, and, it is to be hoped, more efficacious forms of systemic treatment for this disease. At present, administration of chemotherapy to the non-small cell lung cancer patient is entirely appropriate in the context of a controlled clinical trial or on the basis of a well-conceived experimental protocol. In clinical practice, chemotherapy at the present time should be given as "standard therapy" only to patients who are fully ambulatory without other major medical illnesses, who have evaluable tumor lesions so that treatment can be withheld if tumor progression occurs or if response is not forthcoming after several cycles, and who understand the limitations of current treatment, but still desire it.

References

1. Seifter EJ, Ihde DC. Therapy of small cell lung cancer: A perspective on two decades of clinical research. Semin Oncol 1988;15:278–99.
2. Evans WK, Feld R, Osoba D, et al. VP-16 alone and in combination with cisplatin in previously treated patients with small cell lung cancer. Cancer 1984;53:1461–6.
3. Evans WK, Shepherd FA, Feld R, et al. VP-16 and cisplatin as first-line therapy for small cell lung cancer. J Clin Oncol 1985;3:1471–7.
4. Sierocki JS, Hilaris BS, Hopfan S, et al. *cis*-Dichloro-diammine-platinum (II) and VP-16-213: An active induction regimen for small cell carcinoma of the lung. Cancer Treat Rep 1979;63:1593–97.
5. Woods RL, Levi JL. Chemotherapy for small cell lung cancer: A randomized study of maintenance chemotherapy with cyclophosphamide, Adriamycin, and vincristine after remission with cisplatinum, VP-16-213, and radiotherapy. Proc Am Soc Clin Oncol 1984;3:214. Abstract
6. Evans WK, Feld R, Murray N, et al. Superiority of alternating non-cross-resistant chemotherapy in extensive small cell lung cancer. Ann Intern Med 1987;107:451–8.
7. Einhorn LH, Crawford J, Birch R, et al. Cisplatin plus etoposide consolidation following cyclophosphamide, doxorubicin and vincristine in limited small cell lung cancer. J Clin Oncol 1988;6:451–6.
8. Tamura T, Fukuoka M, Furuse K, et al. Japanese multicenter randomized trial: Cyclophosphamide/doxorubicin/vincristine (CAV) versus cisplatin/etoposide (PVP) versus CAV alternating with PVP in patients with small cell lung cancer. Proc Am Soc Clin Oncol 1989;8:220. Abstract
9. Roth BJ, Johnson DH, Greco FA, et al. A Phase III trial of etoposide and cisplatin versus cyclophosphamide, doxorubicin, and vincristine versus alternation of the two therapies for patients with extensive small cell lung cancer. Proc Am Soc Clin Oncol 1989;8:225. Abstract
10. Ihde DC, Johnson BE, Mulshine JL, et al. Randomized trial of high dose versus standard dose etoposide and cisplatin in extensive stage small cell lung cancer. Proc Am Soc Clin Oncol 1987;6:181. Abstract
11. Bunn PA, Ihde DC. Small cell bronchogenic carcinoma: A review of therapeutic results. In: Livingston RB, ed. Lung cancer I. The Hague: Martinus Nijhoff; 1981:169–208
12. Minna JD, Pass H, Glatstein E, et al. Cancer of the lung. In: DeVita VT, Hellman S, Rosenberg SA, eds. Cancer: Principles and practice of oncology, 3rd edn. Philadelphia: JB Lippincott; 1989:591–705.
13. Bunn PA, Lichter AS, Makuch RW, et al. Chemotherapy alone or chemotherapy with chest radiation therapy in limited stage small cell lung cancer: A prospective randomized trial. Ann Intern Med 1987;106:655–62.
14. Feld R, Evans WK, DeBoer G, et al. Combined modality induction therapy without maintenance chemotherapy for small cell carcinoma of the lung. J Clin Oncol 1984;2:294–304.
15. Splinter TAW. EORTC 08825: Induction vs induction plus maintenance chemotherapy in small cell lung cancer: Definitive evaluation. Proc Am Soc Clin Oncol 1988;7:202. Abstract
16. Ettinger DS, Finkelstein DM, Abeloff MD, et al. A randomized comparison of standard chemotherapy versus alternating chemotherapy and maintenance versus no maintenance therapy for extensive stage small cell lung cancer: A Phase III study of the Eastern Cooperative Oncology Group. J Clin Oncol 1990;8:230–40.

17. Evans WK, Osoba D, Feld R, et al. Etoposide (VP-16) and cisplatin: An effective treatment for relapse of small cell lung cancer. J Clin Oncol 1985;3:65–71.
18. Porter LL, Johnson DH, Hainsworth JD, et al. Cisplatin and etoposide combination chemotherapy for refractory small cell carcinoma of the lung. Cancer Treat Rep 1985;69: 479–81.
19. Batist G, Carney DN, Cowan KH, et al. Etoposide (VP-16) and cisplatin in previously treated small cell carcinoma of the lung: Clinical trial and in vitro correlates. J Clin Oncol 1986;4:982–6.
20. Williams CJ, McMillan I, Lea R, et al. Surgery after initial chemotherapy for localized small cell carcinoma of the lung. J Clin Oncol 1987;5:1579–88.
21. Gazdar AF, Steinberg SM, Russell EK, et al. Correlation of in vitro drug sensitivity testing results with response to chemotherapy and survival in extensive stage small cell lung cancer: A prospective clinical trial. J Natl Cancer Inst 1990;82:117–24.
22. Lai SL, Goldstein LJ, Gottesman MM, et al. *MDR*1 gene expression in lung cancer. J Natl Cancer Inst 1989;81:1144–50.
23. Feld R, Rubenstein LV, Weisenberger TH, et al. Sites of recurrence in resected Stage I non-small cell lung cancer: A guide for future studies. J Clin Oncol 1984;2:1352–8.
24. Rapp E, Pater JL, Willan A, et al. Chemotherapy can prolong survival in patients with advanced non-small cell lung cancer: Report of a Canadian multicenter randomized trial. J Clin Oncol 1988;6:633–41.
25. Dillman RO, Seagren SL, Propert K, et al. Protochemotherapy improves survival in regional non-small cell carcinoma. Proc Am Soc Clin Oncol 1988;7:195. Abstract
26. Martini N, Kris MG, Gralla RJ, et al. The effects of preoperative chemotherapy on the resectability of non-small cell carcinoma with mediastinal lymph node metastases (N2M0). Ann Thorac Surg 1988;45:370–9.
27. Lad T, Rubenstein L, Sadeghi A. The benefit of adjuvant treatment for resected locally advanced non-small cell lung cancer. J Clin Oncol 1988;6:9–17.
28. Holmes EC, Gail M. Surgical adjuvant therapy for Stage II and Stage III adenocarcinoma and large undifferentiated carcinoma. J Clin Oncol 1986;4:710–5.

Discussion

Chairperson: **Taisuke Ohnoshi**

Dr Koro Sakoda (Kagoshima Medical Association Hospital, Kagoshima): If a patient has lung cancer in the right upper lobe, accompanied by a small mass in the left upper lobe, possibly due to metastatic cancer, what should we do? Should we operate on him or select some other therapy, such as chemotherapy or immunotherapy?

Dr Ihde: If a patient had 2 apparently surgically resectable diseases, in our institution we would consult our thoracic surgeons immediately and ask them whether this was a patient who might well have 2 primary lung cancers that could be resected. The bronchial tree is like the head and neck mucosa; when you smoke cigarettes the damage is not just restricted to one portion of the mucosa, and simultaneous or synchronous occurrence of 2 primary lung cancers is by no means unheard of. So I would not automatically assume that this patient has metastatic disease and should not undergo surgical resection.

Dr Makoto Ogawa (Cancer Chemotherapy Center, Japanese Foundation for Cancer Research, Tokyo): I would like to know the current understanding of prophylactic cranial irradiation. What is the optimal dose and what are the indications for treatment?

Dr Ihde: Let me first answer for non-small cell lung cancer, since in the USA, at least, there has been some interest in preventive or prophylactic cranial irradiation in this tumor. Data by the Lung Cancer Study Group, looking at carefully staged surgically resected patients for site of first relapse, have established that relapse that is confined to the brain and appears to be confined to the brain for at least 4–6 weeks after the detection of the brain metastases, occurs in only approximately 3% of such patients and therefore one would not expect any benefit from preventive or prophylactic brain irradiation. In small-cell lung cancer there is no question that prophylactic brain irradiation can reduce the frequency of clinical detection of disease in the brain. It appears that this benefit is confined to patients who have a complete response to systemic treatment. This is not surprising because if the patient has only a partial response, the active systemic tumor could metastasize to the brain after the radiation is given.

However, there are worrisome data suggesting that at least some schedules of brain irradiation may be making a major contribution to the neuropsychological impairments that are seen in a fraction of patients with this disease who are long-term survivors. In my own opinion, since there is no suggestion of any survival benefit, I think that, outside of a clinical trial setting, this question should be discussed with the patients and the very unpleasant characteristics of an increased risk of brain metastases or likely impairment of mental function should be discussed with the patient. I think that different patients might well quite reasonably make different decisions when told the facts about the two alternatives, which are both rather depressing.

Dr Nagahiro Saijo (National Cancer Center, Tokyo):   I have 2 questions. One is concerned with the timing of surgery in small cell lung cancer. In highly selective patients, even if chemotherapy is given, before or after surgery, Ginsberg reported that survival in patients receiving chemotherapy before or after surgery is almost the same. In highly selective patients, you stressed that chemotherapy should be given before surgery. I have the same opinion and I would like to reconfirm yours on this point.

Dr Ihde: I think this is a relatively uncommon problem, in the sense that many patients who have initial surgical resection for small cell lung cancer are patients who do not have a preoperative diagnosis of cancer. The patient presents with a small peripheral lesion in which many thoracic surgeons, in North America at least, will proceed directly to operation. So at least in a large fraction of patients who have surgical resection first, one never has the chance to decide whether you might wish to give chemotherapy first. If there is a preoperative diagnosis, I know it is the opinion of many North American thoracic surgeons that chemotherapy should be administered first for the reasons that I outlined. The metastatic disease which is the main determinant of survival is treated first. Secondly, if surgery is of benefit, and I think it is certainly possible that one may well be able to increase the number of patients who are candidates for surgical resection by giving chemotherapy initially, and I agree with that opinion.

Dr Saijo: One more question is about the new drug evaluation in small cell lung cancer. In patients who receive at least one protocol, a more than 10% response rate is permitted for the approval of the drug. Is 10% appropriate or not?

Dr Ihde: Do you think that 10% is a low figure? You are giving investigational drugs after failure of combination chemotherapy, so a high response rate is not to be anticipated, although in certain cases, especially in patients who have not

151

been given chemotherapy for a period of several months, there is a greater likelihood of detecting activity. Nonetheless, the question is, in most diseases you would like to have a 20% response rate before considering that this drug is worth evaluating further, after you have done your phase II study. In small cell lung cancer one approach to selecting new agents is to demand only a 10% response rate in the salvage setting or as 2nd-line treatment and then consider giving that drug a further study. My own feeling is that 10% is close to background noise, in the sense that minor changes in the size of an endobronchial tumor may lead to major changes in atelestasis on chest X ray, for example. I would prefer other strategies. But I recognize that we should have a lower threshold in this situation, because it would be much worse to discard an active drug than to find a drug that was truly inactive and test it some more.

If I could make one other comment about new drug selection, I think a tragedy of the 1980s, which is not restricted to lung cancer, has been that most of the new drugs that have been evaluated were analogues of agents that were already known to be active. Although analogues may have different toxicity profiles that allow a use in unusual situations, such as in intraperitoneal therapy or in very high doses with autologous bone marrow transplant settings, in general I think it is true that an analogue has never really made any major contribution in terms of the antitumor effect compared to the parent drug and I would strongly favor testing drugs that are not analogues of known active agents in this and most other diseases.

Dr Masahiro Fukuoka (Osaka Prefectural Habikino Hospital, Osaka): I would like to ask you about neoadjuvant therapy for non-small cell lung cancer. What stage patients with non-small cell lung cancer should be selected for trials of neoadjuvant chemotherapy followed by surgery?

Dr Ihde: In non-small cell lung cancer there are now numerous pilot studies of giving chemotherapy first, and then attempting surgical resection, some of which are perhaps suggesting survival benefit. I mentioned one that I think is most suggestive, the one by Martini and Gralla from Memorial Sloan-Kettering Cancer Center. Unfortunately, I do not think that any of the studies are conclusive for some of the same reasons that I mentioned in small cell cancer. When one applies historical data, the way in which these tumors are staged has changed over time, with the introduction of CT scans and now MRI scans, meaning that your patients who are now called marginally resectable would have been called operable in the past. There is no question that it is very difficult to get surgeons to agree on who is an operable patient and who is a resectable patient, because, among other things, the surgeons' technical skills will differ and their availability of supporting care in the institution for patients with cardiopulmonary disease varies.

Because of this heterogeneous selection for neoadjuvant chemotherapy in non-small cell lung cancer, I think a prospectively randomized trial is the only way that we can be convinced of the value of this approach. I think that in lung cancer, in contrast to head and neck cancer where local tumor recurrences are a terrible, disfiguring problem, local recurrence is much less frequently a major symptomatic problem that cannot be palliated and survival benefit will need to be shown before neoadjuvant chemotherapy can become standard practice. Simply reducing the rate of local recurrence which would be a very valuable accomplishment in head and neck cancer or bladder or rectal cancer, for example, will not be an appropriate endpoint for deciding that neoadjuvant chemotherapy is proper treatment for lung cancer.

Bone marrow transplantation

Preclinical and clinical considerations in the design of high-dose regimens for solid tumors

Karen H. Antman

Dana-Farber Cancer Institute, Boston, Massachusetts

Introduction

Autologous bone marrow transplantation has proved curative in selected patients with leukemia and lymphoma. Our research is intended to determine whether this technique can be extended to solid tumors such as testicular cancer and breast cancer. We have placed an emphasis on the laboratory considerations in the design of high-dose chemotherapy regimens that require autologous marrow support.

There are 4 criteria for curative bone marrow transplantation, as originally outlined by Santos in 1985 [1]: a malignancy that is responsive to cytoreductive therapy; effective cytoreductive therapy whose dose-limiting toxicity is bone marrow failure; transplant at a time of minimal tumor burden early in the course of the disease when there is the least likelihood of resistance to drugs; and finally, a source of bone marrow stem cells free of clonogenic tumor cells. For leukemia this latter criterion is obviously a major problem and has resulted in the use of allogenic bone marrow when a match is available and investigation into purging techniques when a match is unavailable. For many solid tumors, marrow involvement is not a problem. A source of bone marrow stem cells free of clonogenic tumor cells is available. The major problem for solid tumors is the development of an effective cytoreductive regimen whose limiting toxicity is bone marrow failure.

When trying to design effective regimens for high-dose chemotherapy, laboratory models provide direction since there are many different possible combinations. The strategies can be based on those that were effective in designing curative standard dose treatment for leukemia, lymphoma, and testis cancer. The laboratory models were based on the recognition of the clear linear-log dose-response curve and the observation that combination therapy was necessary because of tumor cell heterogeneity. The use of non-cross-resistant drugs (preferably agents that are synergistic) is optimal.

Combination alkylating agents

The rationale for using combinations of alkylating agents for escalation in transplantation studies is as follows. First, they have broad clinical activity, and second, a steep dose-response curve (reviewed in [2]). At standard doses there is a steep dose-response curve for increasing doses of cyclophosphamide in both sensitive tumors, such as L1210 leukemia, and even in relatively resistant melanoma solid tumors, such as EMT6, in which the slope of the curve is more shallow but remains log linear. The first question to be answered, therefore, was whether this linear log dose-response curve applied to even higher doses, achievable with bone marrow transplant.

In a series of experiments by Teicher et al [3–5], mice with implanted tumors were given the drug or drugs in question at doses increasing into the range achievable with transplant. After 24 h, when all the alkylating activity was completed, the tumor was excised, a cell suspension made, and the tumor cloned. This in vivo, in vitro model was necessary because at these doses most of the animals would die. Using this technique, a steep dose-response curve was found for both cisplatin and carmustine in a fibrosarcoma cell line (Fig 1). This type of

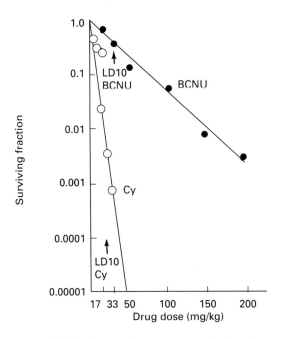

Fig 1 Dose-response curve for high-dose cisplatin and carmustine in a fibrosarcoma LD10 cell line. BCNU, carmustine; Cy, cyclophosphamide. Data from Frei E III et al [6].

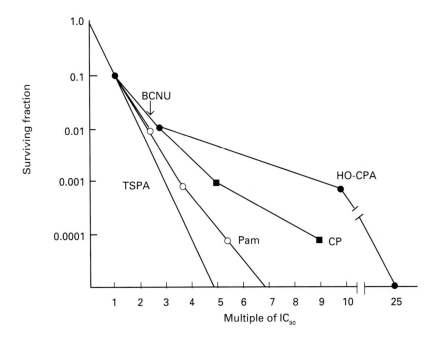

Fig 2 Multilog kill curves: alkylating agents vs breast cancer (MCF7). BCNU, carmustine; HO-CPA, hydroxycyclophosphamide; CP, cisplatin; PAM, melphalan; TSPA, thiotepa. Data from Frei E III et al [6].

model was also used to achieve the results shown in Fig 2. These results are normalized for the dose that results in the first log of tumor cell kill and the doses are expressed as multiplications of the inhibitory constant 90 (IC_{90}). Thiotepa and most of the other alkylating agents shown also followed a steep dose-response curve, although hydroxycyclophosphamide (the activated form of cyclophosphamide) was slightly less effective. However, the laboratory findings were quite different for many of the antimetabolites (Fig 3). After a log or 2 of cell kill there was no advantage in increasing the dose further (except for doxorubicin, however it is difficult to escalate doxorubicin in a transplant setting because of cardiotoxicity). To date, with the exception of etoposide, all the single-agent, high-dose studies have been carried out with alkylating agents.

The degree of escalation that is possible with autologous marrow support is shown in Table 1. For thiotepa the usual standard dose is 30–50 mg/m². The dose can be escalated to about 240 mg without transplant, but Herzig et al [7] have shown that with transplant the dose can be escalated to about 1125 mg, an approximately 38-fold increase in dose. With cyclophosphamide the standard dose is 500 mg/m²; with and without transplant the dose is limited to 7.5 mg because of myopericarditis. Thus an escalation of 10 fold over the standard dose is possible. Mitomycin C, although a good drug for breast cancer at standard doses, cannot be effectively escalated because of the development of venocclu-

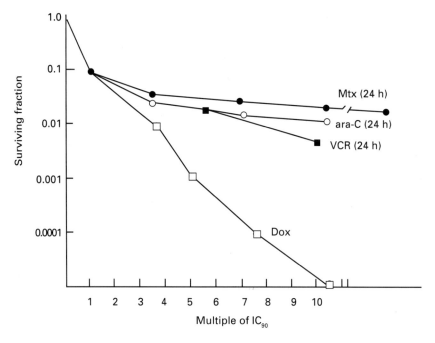

Fig 3 Multilog kill curves: nonalkylating agents vs breast cancer (MCF7). Mtx, methotrexate; ara-C, cytarabine; Dox, doxorubicin. Data from Frei E III et al [6].

sive disease. Cisplatin can be escalated to about 240 mg, but is limited by renal toxicity. Melphalan, however, has been escalated considerably with transplant, as has carmustine. Ifosfamide has been studied in our program. The usual dose is about 5 g/m² and we escalated the dose to 18 g/m², at which point renal toxicity develops [8]. Etoposide has also been escalated to transplant doses. Some of etoposide's effect may be due to its activity as a topoisomerase inhibitor and it may be possible to capitalize on this effect using a relatively standard dose. The advantages of carboplatin over cisplatin are that because of the lack of renal toxicity, carboplatin can be escalated to substantially higher doses than cisplatin; the major toxicity associated with carboplatin has proved to be hepatic, not renal [9].

Another property of alkylating agents is that they tend to be non-cross resistant and also non-cycle specific, unlike antimetabolites; therefore it should be possible to kill cells that are not in cell cycle. It is relatively difficult to achieve resistance to alkylating agents over time by increasing the concentration in tissue culture, whereas it is relatively easy with increasing doses of doxorubicin, or particularly methotrexate, to produce clinical resistance. The kinds of dose escalation that are achievable in the bone marrow transplant setting (4–40 fold) might be capable of overcoming the levels of resistance of 3–15 fold achieved for various alkylating agents.

Most investigators have assumed that alkylating agents will be cross resistant. Schabel has observed that alkylating agents are generally non-cross resistant [2]. Why should alkylating agents be non-cross resistant? They differ substantially in their transport into the cell. Mustard, melphalan, and cisplatin are all actively transported into the cell, but by different transport mechanisms for choline, leucine, and methionine, respectively. Cyclophosphamide, on the other hand, enters the cell via facilitated diffusion, used by the cell for ring compounds, and, finally, the nitrosoureas passively diffuse into the cell. To understand this we need to review the structure of alkylating agents. Most of them have 2 chloroethyl groups, which is basically the structure of mustard. First, an aziridine ring is formed which opens with a covalent bond to one of the strands of DNA. The second chloroethyl group then forms an aziridine ring and either covalently binds onto the other strand or onto the same strand of the DNA, according to the type of alkylating agent; most produce a majority of interstrand DNA cross links. Cisplatin causes intrastrand cross links, dacarbazine only monofunctional links, and procarbazine, basically, DNA breaks. Also the time to the development of the cross link varies from a very short interval for mustard through almost 24 h for cisplatin. When currently available chemotherapeutic agents are classified according to their kinetic effects, most of the antimetabolites and other compounds, such as hydroxyurea and cytarabine, are both cell cycle-specific and proliferation-dependent drugs. However, compounds that are cell-cycle nonspecific but somewhat proliferation dependent tend to be those agents with a fairly long time to cross link, eg, cyclophosphamide and carmustine. Mustard is a drug that is less dependent on cell cycle with a very short time to cross link; the cell does not have sufficient time to repair the damage from the initial link before the cross link occurs.

The alkylating agents, fortunately, have differing organ toxicity at transplant doses. Cyclophosphamide causes a rare but very serious myopericarditis generally at doses above 7 g/m². Melphalan causes mucositis. Carmustine at transplant doses above 600 mg/m² causes pulmonary toxicity (which may occur up to 4–6 months after transplant) and hepatitis or venocclusive disease of the liver. Cisplatin causes renal toxicity. Thiotepa causes mucositis and CNS toxicity. Therefore thiotepa and melphalan, producing the same toxicity, would have little chance of being combined at full transplant doses. These kinds of combinations of agents with the same dose-limiting toxicity should be avoided in the design of high-dose regimens. Mitomycin C results in venocclusive disease and has not often been used in transplants. Carboplatin at high doses results in hepatic and pulmonary toxicity, and ifosfamide, renal and CNS toxicity.

It is interesting that in several experiments, the order of drug administration appears to be significant [4,5,10]. Log cytotoxicity data (Table 1) [10] from the Netherlands using a rat leukemia model and clinical studies using the combination of cyclophosphamide followed by total body irradiotherapy (TBI), showed a clear difference in the relapse rate compared with TBI followed by cyclophosphamide. The situation may be even clearer comparing cyclophosphamide

Table 1 Bone marrow transplantation (BMT) in a rat acute myelogenous leukemia (AML) model: ablative regimens. Data from Hagenbeek A, VanBekkum DW [10].

	BNML log cell kill	% relapse allo-BMT AML 1st CR
Cy/TBI	8.5	25
TBI/Cy	9.5	10
Cy/Bu	10	–
Bu/Cy	>10	0
HDAC + Cy/TBI*	>10	5–10

Cy, cyclophosphamide; Bu, busulfan; CR, complete response; BNML, Brown Norway murine leukemia. *25% treatment-related mortality.

followed by busulfan versus busulfan followed by cyclophosphamide, with the latter being the more effective sequence. Clinicians at Johns Hopkins adopted this order of the combination because busulfan is given by mouth. (When cyclophosphamide is given first emesis prevents administration of the busulfan.) Thus the clinically easier sequence is busulfan followed by cyclophosphamide, which also appears to be the more effective.

So how do the laboratory data apply to the clinic? The majority of institutions currently performing autologous bone marrow transplantation in acute myeloid leukemia (AML) are European. Data were presented in 1989 from France by Gorin [11] on 335 AML patients with a median follow-up of about 2 years. Ten percent of patients had extramedullary leukemia and about 30% received bone marrows that had been purged. The longest follow-up in the European series was for patients transplanted in first complete response. These data appear to show survival superior to that expected with standard treatment. These were highly selected patients, however, and it is difficult to draw conclusions as to whether transplants should be done in first complete response. Although patients transplanted in second complete response have had a much shorter follow-up, it is virtually impossible to cure them with standard treatment and yet some, a respectable 40%, remained disease free at the time that they were analyzed. These are promising data.

High-dose chemotherapy in breast cancer

Which solid tumors would be appropriate to study initially? Obviously, tumors that are invariably fatal with standard treatment, but are extremely sensitive to chemotherapy. Ideal tumors would be breast cancer, small cell lung cancer, and testis cancer. The problem with small cell lung cancer is that these patients are older and have smoked and therefore are at high risk to develop pulmonary toxicity. Early studies are also being done in ovarian cancer, brain tumors, and pediatric sarcomas.

In the USA, about 10% of women develop breast cancer; breast cancer is a much less common disease in Japan, but is increasing in incidence. Two percent of American patients are under age 35 and about 22% under age 55; these could be the candidates for high-dose treatment. If high-dose treatment were safe and effective, it could be extended to women under age 60, which would include half the patients with breast cancer.

First it is important to assess the prognosis for women given standard treatment. We made use of a large database, ie, data from the last 2 randomized trials of the Cancer and Leukemia Group B [12]. Specifically, we wanted to know the prognosis for younger women, who would be candidates for bone marrow transplant. Of the patients who were entered into these 2 trials about half were under age 55, as expected. Interestingly, the treatment mortality was 3.5% for these protocols in patients with stage IV disease. The median remission duration was 8 months and the median survival only 19 months. Women who had had previous adjuvant chemotherapy, liver metastases, or those with estrogen receptor-negative tumors had a particularly poor prognosis. Women with all 3 poor prognostic variables had a median survival of 6 months. For women who were under age 55 with metastatic disease it was considered reasonable and ethical to offer them an experimental treatment.

The rationale for using high-dose therapy in breast cancer is that there does exist a dose response, both experimentally and clinically. The maximum tolerated dose of drugs that are effective in breast cancer is limited by myelosuppression and despite effective palliation, stage IV breast cancer is a fatal disease.

Table 2 is derived from a review of the literature on breast cancer, ranging from single agent studies in women with refractory breast cancer, the worst prognostic group, to combination studies in women who have not received prior treatment for breast cancer, the best prognostic group. There were 4 studies of nonalkylating agents at high dose: 2 with etoposide, 1 with amsacrine, and 1 with hydroxyurea. The total number of women studied was 30. There were no complete responses. Although the patients were progressing through standard treatment, these patients had about a 25% response rate, but the responses were quite

Table 2 Studies of nonalklyating agents in refractory breast cancer. Reprinted, with permission, from Antman KH et al [13].

Author	Drug	g/m	No.	CR	PR	Wk
Mulder	Etoposide	1–1.5	3	0	1	NA
Wolff	Etoposide	1.5–2.7	3	0	0	–
Tannir	Amsacrine	0.6–0.75	16	0	2	18,13
Ariel	Hydroxyurea	40	8	0	3	NA
Total			30	0	6	
%				0	26	

short, measured in terms of weeks, and really of no clinical significance to the patients. There have been more studies of alkylating agents in refractory breast cancer (Table 3): 5 with melphalan, 2 with mitomycin C, 2 with thiotepa, and 1 with high-dose cyclophosphamide. Of the women treated, there was an 11% complete response rate and a 41% overall response rate, but again, with a few notable exceptions, the responses were quite short. This result is expected; in leukemia and in lymphoma studies, when patients are treated with refractory disease, the same kinds of results are obtained. Grouping the studies together, the thiotepa and the melphalan studies were the only agents that produced complete responses. (Almost all these women had been given standard-dose cyclophosphamide prior to the study.)

Table 3 Studies of alkylating agents in refractory breast cancer. Reprinted, with permission, from Antman KH et al [13].

Author	Drug	mg/m	No.	CR	RR	Wk
Knight	Melphalan	180	6	1	4	5–16
Corringham	Melphalan	120	4	3	3	35–94+
Maraninchi	Melphalan	140	4	1	1	24
Lazarus	Melphalan	225	3	0	2	NA
Baker	Melphalan	180	1	0	0	–
Tannir	Mitomycin C	50	15	0	1	<13
Schilcher	Mitomycin C	60	2	0	0	–
LeMaistre	Thiotepa	1575	13	1	8	4 (2–7)
Lazarus	Thiotepa	810	2	0	1	4
Slease	Cyclophosphamide	7800	6	0	3	3,4,8
Total			56	6	23	
%				11	41	

There have also been studies in failed breast cancer with cyclophosphamide and TBI. Only a few women were treated, however, and 3 were in complete response at the time that they were transplanted. (In the Australian study, 2 had had prior liver transplants and 1 had had a lobectomy.) If those 3 patients are excluded, the complete response rate is 29% and the overall response rate 47%.

Combination phase I and phase II studies have been carried out in patients with refractory breast cancer using combinations including cyclophosphamide/carmustine, cyclophosphamide/thiotepa, cyclophosphamide/melphalan, and anthracyclines (Fig 4). Of the total number of women treated, the complete response rate was almost 20% and about 75% of the women responded. In women with refractory disease, however, the durations of response were still quite short. Reviewing the data to assess which drug combinations were most effective, the cyclophosphamide/melphalan combination was found to have the highest complete response rate.

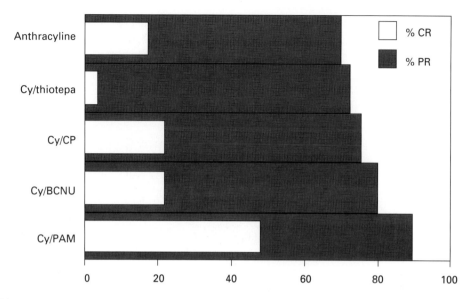

Fig 4 Combination chemotherapy in refractory breast cancer. Cy, cyclophosphamide; CP, cisplatin; BCNU, carmustine.

There have only been 2 studies in patients with no prior treatment treated directly with transplant: one from Duke University and from the Dana-Farber Cancer Institute. Both used cyclophosphamide, carmustine, and cisplatin. In total, 25 women were treated with a comparatively high complete response rate of 56%. The overall response rate was 72%, and 4 (16%) of these women remain continuously in complete response. The woman who has been followed the longest is currently at 61 months, clinically disease free.

Induction therapy

From the data in leukemia and lymphoma, it seems clear that the patients who respond to standard-dose cyclophosphamide are the ones most likely to benefit from high-dose therapy with autologous marrow support. The reasons why an induction therapy might be appropriate are that the tumor burden can be significantly reduced, by perhaps as much as one or two logs. Different drugs can be used to decrease the number of cells resistant to the transplant regimen, or the same drugs to probe for responsive tumors. In lymphoma many patients receive standard-dose chemotherapy and if they respond they are then transplanted with high-dose cyclophosphamide and TBI. However, there are reasons why this strategy might not be effective: it would allow resistant cells to grow during the induction period; multidrug resistance might be induced, although this does not

Table 4 Studies of autologous bone marrow transplantation after induction in previously untreated breast cancer. Reprinted, with permission, from Antman KH et al [13].

Author	Agent	No.	Ind	% CR BMT	CCR	FU (mo)	Deaths
Gisselbrecht	C/TBI	14*	71	86	43	35	0
Livingston	C/TBI	7	29	43	14	30	0
Vaughan	CP or T/TBI	7	43	57	14	20	3
Vincent	L	15	47	80	7	18	3
Russell	L	1	100	100	0	–	0
Maraninchi	CL ± Mitox.	5	80	100	60	10	0
Spitzer	CPE	28	30	71	50	21	2
Jones	CPB	21	52	62	48	13	5
Bitran	CT	22	25	55	14	17	2
Antman	CTCb	10	40	50	50	3	0
Leoni	C/MC/Vb	6	33	67	50	10	0
Total		136		86	47		15
%				68	35		11

*Includes 12 with inflammatory breast cancer (3 stage IV).
C, cyclophosphamide; P, cisplatin; T, thiotepa; L, melphalan; Mitox, mitoxantrone; E, etoposide; B, carmustine; Cb, carboplatin; MC, mitomycin C; Vb, vinblastine.

apply to alkylating agents and so may be a theoretical consideration; or resistance to the alkylating agents might be induced if the same drugs are used later in the transplant.

There are now a number of groups who are studying the treatment of breast cancer with transplant after induction treatment (Table 4). Most of the 136 women entered into these studies have been treated after achieving either a good partial or complete response to prior chemotherapy. The complete response rate has been quite high, as has the partial response rate. Overall the treatment-related death rate varies considerably: the highest mortality is associated with regimens that include carmustine. In our study, 1 patient died of 26 patients entered, so that the mortality is under 4%. However, the overall mortality for all studies was approximately 11%. The single-agent melphalan regimens had a higher complete response rate overall, but they proved to be less durable, suggesting a need for more than one agent. The combination chemotherapy regimens that did not include melphalan had a lower complete response rate, but a more durable response. TBI regimens produced about the same complete response rate, but with slightly more durable responses than regimens that did not include TBI.

To summarize the above data, from the worst prognostic group, ie, those patients with refractory disease treated with single nonalkylating agent chemotherapy to single agent alkylators, combinations that include TBI and combination chemotherapy, untreated patients and responding patients, we can see that

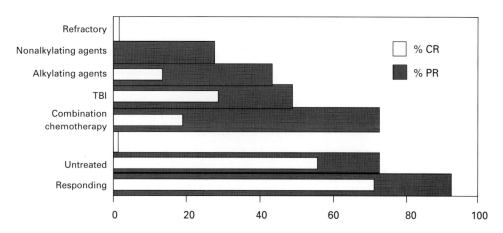

Fig 5   Autologous bone marrow transplantation in breast cancer: summary.

there is a trend toward an increased complete response rate with better risk patients treated with combination therapy (Fig 5).

The future of autologous bone marrow transplantation in breast cancer

For breast cancer, bone marrow transplant is currently expensive. Mortality ranges between 0 and 20% for the various regimens. In refractory disease the remissions are quite short. The optimal preparative regimen is not yet defined, but superior results have been obtained from a variety of regimens in women with less prior treatment, preferably those who are responding to treatment, and with the use of combinations, particularly those including alkylating agents. The response rates with or without TBI appear to be similar and since TBI results in significant toxicity, particularly pulmonary toxicity, it should, perhaps, be avoided.   The role of pretransplant surgery, radiotherapy, or purging of the marrow has yet to be addressed.

There is therefore a dilemma for women who are responding to their first chemotherapy regimen and for their physicians. Transplant yields a high complete response rate, but the percentage of patients who will have durable remissions after high-dose treatment is unknown. Toxic deaths are the least acceptable in this group, but the prognosis for women with stage IV breast cancer is substantially worse than that for a number of other diseases for which some toxic deaths are acceptable. Stage IV disease is an ultimately fatal disease and therefore younger women when faced with the results of standard therapy are frequently willing to participate in these trials.

In our current study, patients receive high doses of doxorubicin (75 mg/m^2

167

over 3 days), fluorouracil (5FU), methotrexate, and leucovorin. Responding patients are restaged and offered bone marrow transplant. Parallel pharmacology is carried out as we are working very close to lethal levels of chemotherapy. After recovery from transplant, any residual disease is resected or radiotherapy is delivered to sites of prior bulk disease. There are 26 patients who have been entered into this trial: 4 are still in the hospital. There are 5 patients who had bone metastases and although their bone scans remain positive (their X rays show sclerosis in those areas), they have responded in all other sites. In this subset of responders, 1 of those 4 has progressed. Of the patients with no bone metastases, 10 have achieved a complete response. There has been 1 toxic death and 1 of the patients has relapsed. The remainder have been disease free for very short intervals from 2 months to a year. Our longest survivor is a patient treated in an earlier study, whose disease-free survival is approximately 6 years.

High-dose chemotherapy in testis cancer

There are now some interesting data accumulating on transplant for testis cancer. The problems in this disease are that patients have often had extensive prior treatment and are often refractory to standard drugs. However they are usually young and generally otherwise healthy, although often they have some renal compromise as a result of prior platinum. Bone marrow involvement is rare (Table 5). The interesting studies to follow are those underway in Indiana, Vancouver, Lyon, and Paris. The total number of patients is still small, but patients in the 2 series of patients in Indiana and Vancouver remain disease free, with a median follow-up of about 1 year. There were some procedure-related deaths in the Indiana series, in which patients received double transplants with high-dose therapies separated by approximately 6 weeks. Nevertheless, since these are patients who had failed after at least 2 prior regimens for testis cancer, they could not have been cured with standard treatment.

Table 5   Studies of high-dose therapy and autologous bone marrow transplantation in refractory testis cancer.

	No.	Rsp	CR	DF	MMFU	PRD
Nichols	33	22	8	5	12	6
Phillips	9		6+	6		0
Biron	7	3	0	0		0
Pico	12	11	3	0	7 (2–16)	2
Total	61	36	17	11		8
%		59	28	18		13

Rsp, response; CR, complete response, DF, disease free; MMFU, median months follow-up; PRD, procedure-related death.

Bone marrow transplantation and hemopoietic growth factors

Finally, autologous bone marrow transplantation has a considerable morbidity and expense. The normal time to neutrophil recovery is 18–26 days after reinfusion. To recover platelets to >20 000/m^3 requires 21–28 days, often longer, and inpatient days are generally at least 39–40. Some patients take a prolonged time for adequate engraftment. Since infection is directly proportional to the duration and depth of neutropenia, virtually all of these patients develop severe infections. There is also a profound psychological effect from prolonged isolation.

Recently, hematopoietic growth factors have become available. Studies have been performed in the transplant setting, particularly with granulocyte-macrophage colony-stimulating factor (GM-CSF) and granulocyte-colony-stimulating factor (G-CSF). Three studies have investigated transplant and GM-CSF; at Duke and Seattle (University of Washington) a significant advantage was shown for patients treated with GM-CSF compared with historical controls. There is a modest difference between the patients who are treated and the historical controls in the Duke study, but a greater difference in the Seattle study (not because the Seattle treatment group did much better, but because the controls were somewhat worse). Interestingly, in the Minnesota study, however, there was no difference between GM-CSF-treated patients and historical controls. These patients were treated with purged marrows while the Duke and Seattle patients did not receive purged marrows, a possible explanation for the negative Minnesota study.

One interesting finding in some of the phase I GM-CSF studies, both in transplants and in standard-dose chemotherapy, is the increase in peripheral blood stem cells when patients are receiving GM-CSF. These data are from our own sarcoma study. With GM-CSF alone there was an approximate 10-fold increase. There was a 2–3-fold increase after chemotherapy alone, but with GM-CSF and chemotherapy during recovery there was up to a 100-fold increase [14]. Many groups have experimented with using peripheral blood stem cells for bone marrow transplants because they are easier to harvest (via techniques for collecting platelets) and there is no need for general anesthesia. Unfortunately, it requires 5–8 leukaphereses currently for adequate stem cell collection and therefore it is technically time-consuming to freeze all of these marrows. On the other hand, with GM-CSF during chemotherapy recovery, it may be possible to collect the required number of peripheral blood stem cells with only one or 2 leukaphereses, if these data are reproducible.

Finally, there is an interesting study going on in breast cancer in Milan [15]. Patients who are eligible with inflammatory breast cancer or 10 or more positive nodes receive cyclophosphamide at 7 g/m^2. A transplant is not needed for this dose. Stem cells are collected on days 14 and 15, the patients then receive further treatment and bone marrow is harvested on day 21. High-dose melphalan therapy is followed by bone marrow and peripheral blood stem cell support. An 8-day

169

median duration of neutropenia has been reported. If this is reproducible, high-dose therapy may become a relatively safe treatment, even for older individuals with cancer. If patients have 8 days of neutropenia after high-dose chemotherapy, they can then be expected to tolerate 2 or perhaps even 3 or 4 sequential treatments and high-dose chemotherapy may become safer, less expensive, and almost standard, since almost any well-trained oncologist can handle the antibiotic needs and the platelet requirement for 8–10 days of neutropenia.

References

1. Santos GW. Overview of autologous bone marrow transplantation. Int J Cell Cloning 1985;3:215–6.
2. Frei E III, Antman K, Teicher B, et al. Bone marrow autotransplantation for solid tumors—prospects. J Clin Oncol 1989;7:515–26.
3. Teicher B, Holden S, Cucchi C, et al. Combination of N, N′, N‴-triethylenethiophosphoramide and cyclophosphamide in vitro and in vivo. Cancer Res 1988;48:94–100.
4. Teicher BA, Holden SA, Eder JP, et al. Influence of schedule on alkylating agent cytotoxicity in vitro and in vivo. Cancer Res 1989;49:5994–8.
5. Teicher BA, Holden SA, Jones SM, et al. Influence of scheduling on two-drug combinations of alkylating agents in vivo. Cancer Chemother Pharmacol. In press.
6. Frei E, Teicher BA, Holden SA, et al. Preclinical studies and clinical correlation of the effect of alkylating dose. Cancer Res 1988;48:6417–23.
7. Herzig RH, Fay JW, Herzig GP, et al. Phase I–II studies with high-dose thiotepa and autologous marrow transplantation in patients with refractory malignancies. In: Herzig GP, ed. Advances in cancer chemotherapy: high dose thiotepa and autologous marrow transplantation. Park Row; 1987:17–33.
8. Elias A, Eder JP, Shea T, et al. High-dose ifosfamide with mesna uroprotection: A phase I study. J Clin Oncol 1990;8:170–8.
9. Shea TC, Flaherty M, Elias A, et al. A phase I clinical and pharmacological study of high-dose carboplatin and autologous bone marrow support. J Clin Oncol 1989;7:651–61.
10. Hagenbeek A, VanBekkum DW. Proceedings of a workshop on comparative evaluation of the L5222 and the BAL rat leukaemia models and their relevance for human acute leukaemia. Leukemia Res 1977;1:75–255.
11. Gorin N, Aegerter P, Auvert B. Autologous bone marrow transplantation (ABMT) for acute leukaemia in remission. An analysis on 1322 cases. Bone Marrow Transpl 1989;4:3–5.
12. Mick R, Begg CB, Antman K, et al. Diverse prognosis in metastatic breast cancer. Who should be offered alternative initial therapies? Breast Cancer Res Treat 1989;13:33-8.
13. Antman KH, Eder JP, Elias E, et al. High dose chemotherapy in breast cancer. In: Ariel IM, Ragaz J, eds. High risk breast cancer. New York:Springer-Verlag. In press.
14. Socinski MA, Cannistra SA, Elias A, et al. Granulocyte macrophage colony stimulating factor expands the circulating haemopoietic progenitor cell compartment in man. Lancet 1988;i:1194–8.
15. Gianni AM, Bregni M, Siena S, et al. Rapid and complete hematopoietic reconstitution following combined transplantation of autologous blood and bone marrow cells. A changing role for high dose chemoradiotherapy. Hemat Oncol 1989;7:139–48.
16. Goldstone AH, Gribben JG, McMillan AK, Taghipour G. The sixth report of the EBMTG

registry for ABMT in lymphoma. Bone Marrow Transplant 1989;4(Suppl 2):53.

17. Sharp J, Armitage J, Crouse D, et al. Recent progress in the detection of metastatic tumor in bone marrow by culture techniques. In: Dicke K, Spitzer G, Jagannath S, Evinger-Hodges M, eds. Autologous bone marrow transplantation, proceedings of the fourth international symposium. Houston: University of Texas MD Anderson Cancer Center Press; 1989;421–7.

18. Mulder P, Willemse P, Aalders JG, et al. High-dose chemotherapy with autologous bone marrow transplantation in patients with refractory ovarian cancer. Eur J Cancer Clin Oncol 1988;25:645–9.

19. Stoppa AM, Maraninchi D, Niens P, et al. High doses of melphalan and autologous marrow rescue in advanced common epithelial ovarian carcinomas: A retrospective analysis in 35 patients. In: Dicke K, Spitzer G, Jagannath S, Evinger-Hodges MJ, eds. Autologous bone marrow transplantation. Houston: University of Texas MD Anderson Cancer Center; 1989:509–18.

20. Gabrilove JL, Jakubowski A, Scher H, et al. Effect of granulocyte colony-stimulating factor on neutropenia and associated morbidity due to chemotherapy for transitional-cell carcinoma of the urothelium. N Engl J Med 1988;318:1414–22.

Discussion

Chairperson: **Tomoo Tajima**

Dr Hiroshi Fujita (Tsurumi University School of Dental Medicine, Yokohama): I understand that high-dose chemotherapy and bone marrow transplantation result in a very high CR rate. However, in Japan, toxic death is regarded as a very serious problem, even when the incidence is less than 10%. I wonder whether it is appropriate to give alkylating agents at the high doses you recommended to patients with markedly reduced hepatic or renal function? Alkylating agents are detoxified in these organs. For example, can one give cisplatin to patients with renal disorders? Also, bone marrow rescues patients from bone marrow toxicity, but not from other toxicities. For instance, mitomycin C at a dose of 50–60 mg/m^2 is very toxic to the liver. I think such a dose is dangerous. I believe that in order to reduce the incidence of toxic deaths associated with these high doses, the blood levels of these agents should be monitored in each patient and a detoxifying agent, such as sodium thiosulfate in the case of cisplatin, should be given when a high blood level has been recorded over a long period. What is your view on this?

Dr Antman: First, I agree that in general a high mortality is unacceptable, unless it has been proven that this is curative treatment for most people. If 50–60% of people patients are cured with standard treatment, then I find a 20% mortality acceptable. With our current regimen we have about a 4% mortality, which is not significantly different from the 3.5% seen from the CALGB standard-dose trial. The reason that we took an extra year or 2 to develop the cyclophosphamide/thiotepa regimen was that we found the cyclophosphamide/carmustine regimen to be too toxic. We tried to change the schedule to avoid the venocclusive disease and other toxicities, but we could not decrease the mortality, so we developed another regimen.

Regarding your second question: how does one treat patients with underlying kidney or liver compromise? When those are caused by cancer, probably the best technique is to try to control the tumor with standard-dose treatment. When the liver function tests are as good as possible, transplant will be safer. The incidence of venocclusive disease is significantly associated with underlying liver disease, such as an elevated SGOT or hepatitis. Therefore we do not transplant patients with significantly elevated liver function tests. For the patients with renal toxicity (such as patients with testis cancer who have had prior platinum) we are

172

trying to design a regimen with minimal kidney toxicity using high doses of carboplatin, which has no renal toxicity. On the other hand, patients with testis cancer have a uniformly fatal disease by the time transplant is considered and some compromise of their renal function is probably worthwhile, if one could cure 15%, as the Indiana data suggest is possible.

Dr Makoto Ogawa (Cancer Chemotherapy Center, Japanese Foundation for Cancer Research, Tokyo): I would like to know the role of total body irradiation (TBI) in the case of lymphoma. We understand that TBI is not necessary for advanced breast cancer, however what about non-Hodgkin lymphoma? My second question is that I was surprised to hear that mitomycin C can be administered at a dose of 90 mg/m², which is a very high dose compared to the previous report from Wayne State University. Can you give us any further information, because if it is possible, we can apply it to other tumors?

Dr Antman: Most of the original transplants in non-Hodgkin lymphoma were done with cyclophosphamide/TBI. I am not aware of a significant difference in these data between patients who received TBI and those who received combination chemotherapy. For the Hodgkin disease patients who received radiotherapy there was double the mortality [16]. Probably the difference is that the Hodgkin patients have received prior mantle radiotherapy and they had have more pulmonary deaths. So there was a significant difference between those who received chemotherapy-only regimens, with a mortality of 11% and 22% in the Hodgkin patients who received the TBI regimen.

The second question was about mitomycin C. The 2 groups that were treated in the mitomycin C phase I trials did get to 90 mg/m², but with unacceptable toxicity. There was a substantial mortality from venoocclusive disease in the one study and severe mucositis and diarrhea in the other study, so both groups abandoned mitomycin C.

Dr Tomoo Tajima (Tokai University School of Medicine, Isehara): I would like to confirm the current role of TBI in lymphoma. Do you think there is a place for TBI?

Dr Antman: In non-Hodgkin lymphoma, the mortality, response rate, and duration of survival were not different for those who received the chemotherapy-alone regimen or for those who received the TBI regimen. For Hodgkin disease there was a substantial increase in the mortality for those who received the TBI regimen.

Dr Tajima: How about the usual surgical solid tumor? Do you think there is a place for TBI?

Dr Antman: For breast cancer, probably not for TBI at this time, but there probably will be a place for radiating prior sites of bulk disease.

Dr Yutaka Tokuda (Tokai University School of Medicine, Isehara): I would like to ask a question about peripheral blood stem cell transfusion. This technique is very promising, especially for breast cancer, because breast cancer patients often have contamination of the bone marrow with tumor cells. However, all the studies from Australia reveal that after injection of peripheral blood stem cells, patients often experience prolonged thrombocytopenia. Do you have any data about in vitro assays of progenitor cells for platelets in the peripheral blood stem cells?

Dr Antman: I have no data on CFU for megakaryocytes However, it has been found that the number of peripheral blood stem cells that have to be reengrafted is about 10–100 times the number of CFU-GM needed for bone marrow. The original studies from Australia and from Europe looking at peripheral blood stem cell transplants used the same number of CFU-GM as they would have used for bone marrow and they had very poor engraftment, particularly of platelets. Those same groups found in more recent trials with adequate numbers of CFU-GM show a day or 2 slower recovery of platelets than of neutrophils, but adequate engraftment. Clearly the CFU-GM and bone marrow and the CFU-GM and peripheral blood are somewhat different.

Dr Tajima: To follow on from Dr Antman's answer, we recently checked the bone marrow, different kinds of progenitor cells, and the CFU in the megakaryocyte lineage appeared to be the most vulnerable to changes from outside.

Dr Antman: I think you are right, because all of the groups have reported slower platelet recovery than of neutrophils using support from either bone marrow or peripheral blood.

Dr Taketo Mukaiyama (Cancer Chemotherapy Center, Japanese Foundation for Cancer Research, Tokyo): I have 2 questions. First, I would like to know what you think about maintenance chemotherapy after high-dose chemotherapy, and second, do you have any ideas on accelerating the recovery of cellular immunity using cytokines or drugs?

Dr Antman: To take the second question first, about accelerating recovery, we (and probably you and others) see about one year of inverted T cell markers after autologous bone marrow transplant. We have not done any experiments to increase the immunological recovery. Clinically, the only thing that we have seen is the development of shingles in about 10% of the patients. We are thinking of trying prophylactic aciclovir in those patients, but since clinically it does not seem to be much of a problem, we have not done any experiments with biologicals to increase the recovery.

To answer your other question, most patients after bone marrow transplants relapse and they still have to be treated. These patients can receive chemotherapy if they relapse 6 months or more after their transplant and it is possible to give almost full-dose treatment. We have not tried maintenance treatment after bone marrow transplant, but from the data in patients who relapse, it should be possible.

Dr Yoichi Takaue (University of Tokushima School of Medicine, Tokushima): Back to the issue of peripheral blood stem cell transplantation, I would like to add a question and comment based on our other study. We have so far treated 15 patients and all were grafted with circulating stem cells. However, the point I want to address is that we only need a couple of leukaphereses. In such a case, I wonder whether the use of this procedure up front in the treatment of patients with leukemia or lymphoma can be justified or not. That is my question. My comment is on the issue of contamination by clonogenic leukemic or tumor cells. So far we have not seen any suspicious cases of early relapse, due to contaminated clonogenic leukemic cells or other cells like neuroblastoma cells. So I think we can apply this procedure safely and even extend it to the treatment of a variety of cancers. We believe that the mere presence of malignant cells in the circulation per se does not preclude the possibility of performing this procedure.

Dr Antman: I think your comments are very well taken. When tumor involves the bone marrow, it clearly is clonogenic, growing there. The tumor cells that may circulate in the peripheral blood may not be necessarily clonogenic. It is well known that during mastectomy cancer cells circulate in the buffy coat. Yet that has no significance as to whether or not the woman will relapse after mastectomy. So clearly the tumor cells that circulate, at least in breast cancer, may not be clonogenic. The group who have data to address this is at Nebraska, where they have attempted to grow tumors from bone marrow harvests. In bone marrows that are histologically negative malignant-appearing cells have grown [17]. When they used peripheral blood stem cells they have not yet been able to

175

grow clonogenic tumor cells from the marrow. So, for as yet unknown reasons, peripheral blood may be a better source of stem cells.

Dr Tajima: So this approach would represent a quite promising future direction?

Dr Antman: Yes.

Dr Haruhiko Dozono (Kagoshima University School of Medicine, Kagoshima): I have 2 questions. First, if bone marrow transplantation is used in ovarian cancer, what type of agents should be given, and to what extent? Second, if, for example, methotrexate is given at high doses, stomatitis may occur. Do you give supportive therapy in such cases?

Dr Antman: In ovarian cancer only 2 groups have reported a significant number of patients with transplants [18,19]. In a phase II study some patients remain in complete response with short periods of follow-up. I do not know whether or not this will be an effective treatment.

Your other question was mucositis related to methotrexate. Certainly the regimens that we have been using in breast cancer (doxorubicin, methotrexate, and fluorouracil) resulted in significant mucositis. We are about to start a study that will give GM-CSF after each course. We are hoping that the observation made by the group at Memorial Sloan-Kettering Institute [20], that the mucositis will be reduced by GM-CSF and allow us to deliver the treatment on time. I do not know of any other prophylactic against mucositis than the possibility of G-CSF or GM-CSF.

Dr Tajima: I would like to ask a final question about the nomenclature of ABMT. We have been using the terms "transplantation," "autotransplantation," "marrow rescue," and "reinfusion." Which do you prefer?

Dr Antman: Scientifically, it is support. Autologous bone marrow transplant is not really an organ transplant, it is a sophisticated support mechanism that allows the physician to give substantially higher doses of chemotherapy and therefore, scientifically, we should be discussing autologous marrow support, but it is easier to use "autotransplant" or "AMBT" when speaking.

Author index